K. Eguchi, J. Klastersky, R. Feld (Eds.)

Current Perspectives and Future Directions in
Palliative Medicine

With 20 Figures

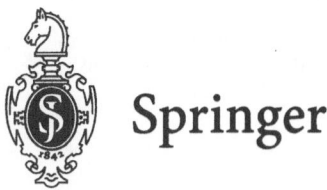

Springer

Kenji Eguchi
Vice Director, National Shikoku Cancer Center
13 Horinouchi, Matsuyama, Ehime 790-8501, Japan

Jean Klastersky
Professor and Chief of Medicine, Institut Jules Bordet
Centre des Tumeurs de l'Université Libre de Bruxelles
Bruxelles, Rue Héger-Bordet 1, 1000, Bruxelles, Belgique

Ronald Feld
Professor of Medicine, Ontario Cancer Institute/Princess Margaret Hospital
610 University Ave., Toronto, Ontario, Canada M5G 2M9

ISBN-13: 978-4-431-68496-1   e-ISBN-13: 978-4-431-68494-7
DOI: 10.1007/978-4-431-68494-7

Printed on acid-free paper

Typesetting: Camera-ready by authors

SPIN: 10688305

PREFACE

"Evidence-based management" has become an important issue for palliative medicine in patients with incurable diseases, such as relapsed cancers, acquired immunodeficiency sydrome (AIDS), and chronic progressive neurologic disorders. For this reason, "The International Symposium on Current Perspectives and Future Directions in Palliative Medicine 1997," organized by the Japan Intractable Diseases Research Foundation with the support of the Japanese Ministry of Health and Welfare, was held at the International Lecture Hall of the National Cancer Center, Tokyo on October 29 and 30, 1997. The goal of this symposium was to present health professionals with a multidisciplinary approach to improve comprehensive palliative care.

The program prepared by the Organizing Committee and the International Organizing Committee (Prof. Jean Klastersky, Prof. Ronald Feld, and myself) focused on the following topics: standard management and clinical trials for controlling such symptoms as pain, cachexia, intestinal obstruction, chronic nausea and vomiting, neutropenic infection, and dyspnea; management of depression; ethics in palliative medicine; health economics; quality of life (QOL) research; and patient education. Twenty speakers -- 5 from the USA, 3 from Canada, 1 from the Netherlands, 1 from Belgium, and 10 from Japan -- presented results of their recent investigations. In addition, more than 180 specialists from areas related to palliative medicine participated in this symposium. Extensive and lively discussions were held after each lecture to identify areas of controversy, to describe recent advances in therapy, to predict future approaches to management, to update new research techniques, and to explore and resolve major subjects of disagreement.

Increased understanding of the fundamental mechanisms of symptoms in patients with advanced cancer, AIDS, and other incurable diseases is urgently needed. Furthermore, available information must be integrated so that obstacles to better palliation can be overcome. Collaborative work in palliative medicine should be expanded to multinational study groups. I hope the results of this symposium will set new standards and provide new perspectives for clinical practice and research in palliative medicine for patients suffering from incurable diseases.

I wish to express my gratitude to the invited speakers who generously honored us with their sincere and friendly participation. My thanks also go to the discussants who contributed to the success of the symposium. I wish to thank the other members of the organizing committee, Prof. Jean Klastersky, Prof. Ronald Feld, Prof. Kaoru Abe, Prof. Fumimaro Takaku, and Prof. Tetsuichiro Mutou, whose sincere support and advice helped make this symposium a success.

The Organizing Committee is grateful to the Japan Intractable Diseases Research Foundation, and in particular, to Mr. Kenji Yoshihara, Mr. Naofumi Fukai, and Ms. Shukue Azuma. We would also like to express our sincere thanks to Dr. Hiroki Nakatani, Dr. Taro Tsukahara, and Dr. Atsuhiro Mitsumaru of the Japanese Ministry of Health and Welfare for their support of this symposium. It is a great pleasure for me to extend my sincere thanks to Ms. Keiko Iwadate and Ms. Ayumi Okimoto for their secretarial work. Finally, we would like to thank the staff of Springer-Verlag Tokyo for their extensive help in the preparation of this publication.

Kenji Eguchi, MD
Chairman of the Organizing Committee

ORGANIZATION OF SYMPOSIUM

SYMPOSIUM COMMITTEE

Japan Intractable Diseases Research Foundation

CHAIRMAN

Kenji Eguchi	Vice Director National Shikoku Cancer Center, Matsuyama, Japan

INTERNATIONAL ORGANIZING COMMITTEE

Jean Klastersky	Professor and Chief of Medicine Institut Jules Bordet, Bruxelles, Belgium
Ronald Feld	Professor of Medicine Ontario Cancer Institute / Princess Margaret Hospital Toronto, Canada

LOCAL ORGANIZING COMMITTEE

Kaoru Abe	President, National Cancer Center, Tokyo
Satoshi Ebihara	Director, National Cancer Center Hospital East, Kashiwa
Nobuyoshi Fukuhara	Vice Director, National Saigata Hospital, Niigata
Kazuaki Hiraga	Chief, National Cancer Center Hospital, Tokyo
Kunihiko Ishitani	Director, Higashi Sapporo Hospital, Sapporo
Hideaki Nagai	Chief, National Tokyo Hospital, Tokyo
Nasayoshi Negishi	Chief, Department of Infectious Disease Tokyo Metropolitan Komagome Hospital, Tokyo
Nagashiro Saijo	Chief, National Cancer Center Research Institute, Tokyo
Yasuo Shima	Head, Palliative Care Unit, National Cancer Center Hospital East, Kashiwa
Fumimaro Takaku	President, Jichi Medical School, Tochigi
Fumikazu Takeda	President, Saitama Cancer Center, Saitama
Toru Watanabe	Head, Department of Internal Medicine National Cancer Center Hospital, Tokyo
Fumiko Yamanishi	Deputy Manager, Guidance Section of Nurse Training Schools, Division of Hospital Service Policy, Department of National Hospitals, Health Service Bureau Ministry of Health and Welfare, Tokyo
Shigeto Yamawaki	Professor and Chairman, Department of Psychiatry and Neurosciences, Hiroshima University, School of Medicine, Hiroshima

ACKNOWLEDGEMENTS

The editors gratefully acknowledge the support of the following organizations and individuals.

HOST ORGANIZATIONS

The Japan Intractable Diseases Research Foundation
The Japanese Ministry of Health and Welfare

SECRETARY-GENERAL

Shukue Azuma

TABLE OF CONTENTS

LIST OF AUTHORS

Session I

Symptom Control in Palliative Medicine:
Standard Management and Clinical Trials I

Chairpersons:
Jean Klastersky and Kenji Eguchi

RECENT RESEARCH IN PAIN AND CACHEXIA IN ADVANCED CANCER AND AIDS

Eduardo Bruera

Professor of Oncology, Alberta Cancer Foundation Chair in Palliative Medicine, Grey Nuns Community Hospital & Health Centre, Edmonton, AB Canada

SUMMARY

During recent years there have been major developments in the assessment and management of pain and cachexia in patients with advanced cancer. Many of these developments are applicable to patients with other terminal conditions including AIDS. A number of researchers have emphasized the need for a appropriate assessment and monitoring of the intensity of multiple symptoms. A number of predictors of outcome have been recently recognized, including neuropathic pain, incidental pain, tolerance, history of alcoholism or drug addiction, and somatization. As a result of increased education patients are receiving higher doses of opioids for cancer pain. This has brought increased understanding on the neurotoxicity of opioids, including delirium, hallucinations, myoclonus, hyperalgesia, and grand mal seizures. Both the parent compounds and multiple metabolites have been associated with these side effects. During recent years a number of clinical trials have confirmed the role of prokinetic agents, progestational drugs, and corticosteroids in the management of cancer cachexia. In addition, a group of new and exciting drugs are undergoing research including thalidomide, melatonin, and clenbuteral.

KEY WORDS: Cancer, cachexia, nutrition, pain, opioids, assessment

INTRODUCTION

Approximately 50% of patients diagnosed with cancer will die because of progressive disease [1]. Pain and cachexia are among the most frequent and devastating symptoms in these patients.

During the last five years, two of the major developments in cancer pain have been an increased understanding on the importance of careful multidimensional assessment, and improved characterization of opioid-induced neuropsychiatric effects. In the area of cachexia, after many years of limited development, a number of exciting new agents are currently undergoing clinical trials.

The purpose of this paper is to review some of these developments. Most of the information on palliative interventions has been acquired in clinical trials on cancer patients. However, the concepts regarding assessment, neuropsychiatric effects, and pharamcological interventions for cachexia are generally applicable to patients with the devastating complications associated with advanced and terminal AIDS.

MULTIDIMENSIONAL ASSESSMENT IN PALLIATIVE CARE

Figure 1 summarizes the different components of the symptom experience. The production of a symptom is the process by which nociception occurs at the level of a primary or metastatic tumor site in the case of pain, or afferent stimulation of the "j" receptors take place in the case of dyspnea. The production can be significantly different from one individual to another and in different areas within the same individual (eg: some patients have multiple bone metastases of which only one hurts). Unfortunately, the process of production cannot be measured clinically. Perception is the process by which the symptom reaches the brain cortex. This can also have significant variation over time and among different individuals. Some modulating factors for the perception of symptoms are well known, such as endorphins or descending inhibitory pathways in the case of pain. Unfortunately, perception cannot be measured. Finally, the expression of the distress is the only clinically measurable part of the experience and is the target of all treatment interventions. However, this stage can also be very variable from one individual to another due to beliefs about the symptom experience, intra-psychic factors such as depression or somatization, and even cultural factors. The different symptomatic interventions are then addressed to the three components of the symptom experience. In the case of pain, treatments such as radiation therapy are aimed towards decreasing the production of nociception, treatments such as opioid therapy attempt to decrease perception, and the management of psychosocial distress and delirium attempt to decrease the expression of distress.

In summary, while it is very important to measure the intensity of a certain symptom such as pain or nausea, it is important to recognize that the intensity of expression does not have the same unidimensional value of the blood glucose in the case of the control of diabetes, or the blood pressure in the case of the control of arterial hypertension. Interpreting the intensity of the pain expression as being only the expression of nociception would deny that in addition to variability in nociception, there is a great variability in both perception and expression of pain. Rather, pain expression should be interpreted as a multidimensional construct. While two patients might express an identical pain intensity of 8 out of 10, in one of the cases, the expression may be almost completely due to nociception, while in the other case, factors such as opioid development of tolerance, somatization, or depression might have great impact on the symptom expression. The multidimensional assessment should help in the recognition of the contribution of the different dimension to the patient's expression, and thereby, assist the planning of appropriate care. A purely unidimensional interpretation of the intensity of pain would result in assuming that 100% success can be achieved with a simple use of higher doses of analgesics. This simplistic approach could result in massive doses of opioids, opioid related toxicity, and excessive reliance on pharmacological as compared to non-pharmacological approaches to symptom control. A number of tools can be used in order to assess the contribution of different dimensions to the patient's symptom expression.

Figure 1:   Components of the Symptom Experience

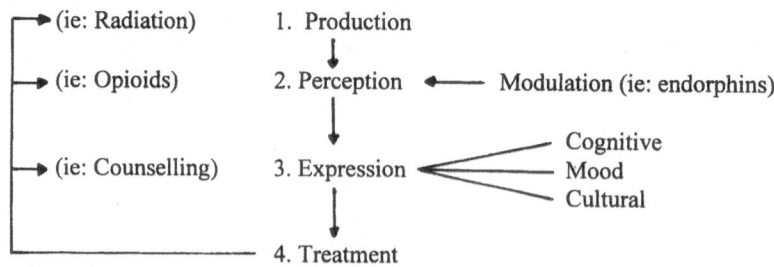

Edmonton Symptom Assessment System (ESAS)

This system consists of nine different visual analogue scales that assess nine different symptoms. In patients who are unable to complete the visual analogue scale, the intensity of the symptom can be reported verbally as a number that is then recorded by the nurse or relative. The results, in terms of symptom intensity, can then be recorded in a graphic display in the patient's chart (Figure 2). This allows for follow-up on a daily basis on admitted patients and also to compare changes in symptoms between visits of patients at home. While most patients are able to complete their own assessment during the beginning of the treatment, in almost all cases, the assessment needs to be completed by the nurse or relative during the last days of life [2]. The ESAS is useful in the initial assessment at follow-up of different symptom complexes. It allows for the interpretation of visual patterns associated with the predominance of physical or psychosocial symptoms. It also allows the team to discuss with the patients the meaning of the high intensity of expression of a given symptom when the patient's verbal description during rounds, drug take or behavior in-between assessments is not consistent with the intensity of the symptom complaint. Finally, the ESAS can also be used for quality control by documenting the characteristics of patients admitted to different areas of a comprehensive palliative care program. Ideally, patients admitted to a tertiary palliative care unit should have an overall high intensity in the ESAS as compared to patients admitted to long-term care wards or those managed at home.

In different areas of the world, a large number of tools have been used for the assessment of the intensity of different symptoms [3-10]. These tools utilize descriptions of intensity using numbers, words, fingers on the hand, or pointing at circles of different size or color. All these systems appear to be quite reliable in the assessment of the intensity of different symptoms. One important consideration is that the intensity of symptoms be appropriately recorded and monitored so as to allow for appropriate monitoring of symptom intensity of time.

Figure 2:   Symptom Assessment Forms

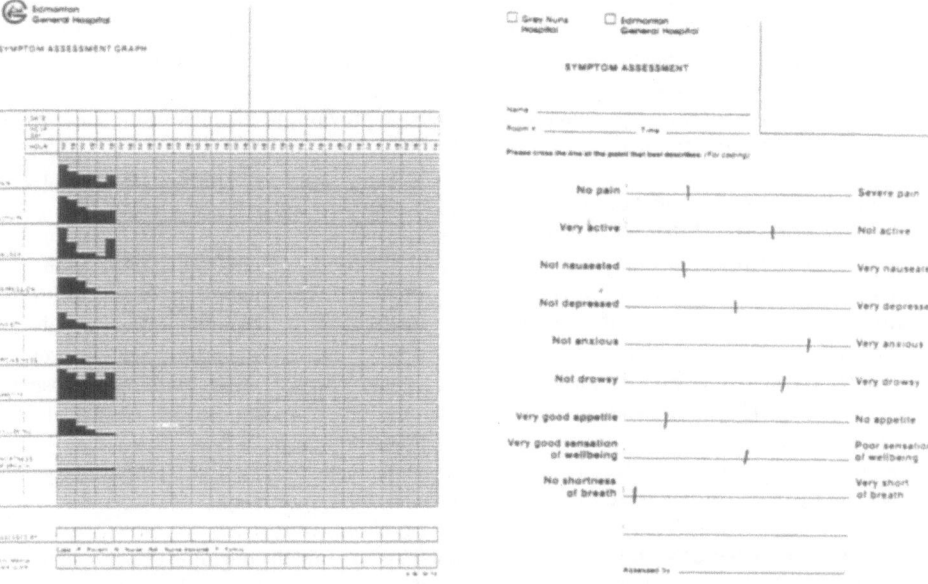

Edmonton Staging System for Cancer Pain

This system assesses five major clinical features that have been found to have prognostic implications in patients treated with systemic analgesics and adjuvant drugs (table 1).

Table 1: New Staging System

Stage 1:	Good prognosis	
	A1 (Visceral)	
	F1 (No tolerance)	
	A2 (Bone/soft tissue)	
	B1 (Non-incidental)	
	E1 (No somatization)	
	G1 (No alcohol/drugs)	
Stage 2:	Poor prognosis	
	A3 (Neuropathic)	(Any B-E-F-G)
	A4 (Mixed)	(Any B-E-F-G)
	A5 (Unknown)	(Any B-E-F-G)
	B2 (Incidental)	(Any A-E-F-G)
	E2 (Somatization)	(Any A-B-F-G)
	F2 (Tolerance)	(Any A-B-E-G)
	G2 (Alcohol/drugs)	(Any A-B-E-F)

After an initial consultation, the treating physician is able to complete a simple form including these prognostic in less than five minutes. The staging system considers the following items:

1. *Mechanism of pain (a)*. Visceral and bone/soft tissue pain syndromes are considered to be associated with good prognosis, while pain of neuropathic, mixed or unknown origin is considered an indication of poor prognosis.
2. *Pain characteristics (b)*. Pain of mild intensity addressed and of severe and excruciating intensity during movements, swallowing, defecation or urination is associated with poor response to analgesics.
3. *Presence of somatization (e)*. Somatization related to previous personality of the presence of mood disorders (eg: depression) is associated with poor prognosis.
4. *Tolerance (f)*. The classification considers the presence of tolerance (need to increase about more than 5% of the initial dose of opioid/day) as poorly prognostic, and the lack of tolerance (less than 5% increase/day) as associated with good prognosis.
5. *History of alcohol or drug dependence (g)*. A past history of addictive personality, with demonstrated addiction to alcohol or drugs may predispose patients to cope chemically with psychological distress, even if the opioid drugs are given for the treatment of cancer pain. Patients are considered to have good prognosis if they have no history or alcohol or drug addiction and to have poor prognosis if there is a positive history. After an initial assessment in 52 patients [11], a multicenter study was conducted in 277 patients [12]. Of 276 evaluable patients, 86/92 Stage I patients achieved good pain control during a final assessment on day 21 (23%) versus 102/185 Stage II (poor prognosis) patients, 55% (p<0.001). Sensitivity and specificity of the system were found to be 0.93 and 0.46, respectively.

The present data suggests that this system is accurate in predicting the outcome of patients with good prognosis. However, patients with more difficult pain syndromes can still achieve good pain control in almost half of the cases. These results are similar to those of other screening instruments such as the bone scan for the detection of bone metastases. While accuracy of this staging system could be improved, the present data suggests that this is a simple and reliable instrument that might allow for better planning in the care of these patients and for better description of the characteristics of patients admitted to different clinical trials.

Mini-Mental State Questionnaire

Most cancer patients develop severe cognitive failure before death [13]. Unfortunately, physicians and nurses frequently fail to detect cognitive failure in these patients [13]. To detect cognitive impairment, various screening tests have been developed [14] including the Mini-mental state examination (MMSE) and the Blessed Orientation Memory Concentration test (BOMC). The MMSE has been utilized and tested extensively in patients with cancer [14]. It is a simple tool that requires only a few minutes to administer and can easily be performed by minimally trained caregivers. Frequent administration of the MMSE have been found to be useful in following up patient sin palliative care settings [15]. In addition, a recent retrospective study suggests that improvement of cognition as indicated by normalization of an MMSE correlates with an increased discharge rate from a palliative care unit [15].

The screening tools discussed above are sensitive indicators of cognitive impairment, but are not specific for the diagnosis of delirium. In addtion, they do not quantify the severity of delirium and do not provide a phenomenology of delirium. Several instruments have been developed and validated to facilitate the specific diagnosis of delirium [14]. These tools cannot be applied repeatedly and are able to monitor short-term changes. The Memorial Delirium Assessment Scale (MDAS) has been developed more recently as a method of quantifying the severity of delirium on a frequent basis [15]. It appears to have diagnostic properties as well.

The Assessment of Alcohol and Drug Abuse

A history of alcoholism or drug abuse has been identified to be an independent prognostic factor for poor pain control. These patients, when faced with life stressors, tend to utilize maladaptive coping strategies. Despite the relatively high frequency of alcoholism in the general population, a recent study suggests that physicians from different specialties missed the diagnosis of alcoholism in the great majority of patients under their care during a hospital admission [16]. This study utilized the CAGE screening questionnaire. The four key questions in this questionnaire include: a) has the patient ever been asked to "cut back" on alcohol intake; b) ever "annoyed" by people suggesting alcohol avoidance; c) ever felt "guilty" about alcohol consumption, and d) did he/she ever require an "eye opening" drink in the morning [17]. Although classified as a screening tool, the CAGE questionnaire can predict with a high level of specificity and sensitivity the presence of alcoholism in patients who score positively for two or more of the questions. When the CAGE questionnaire was utilized in consecutive admissions to a tertiary palliative care unit, the prevalence was found to be 27%. The combination of intensive counseling with pharmacological management of cancer pain resulted in overall pain control and analgesic consumption that were comparable between alcoholic and non-alcoholic patients with cancer pain [17]. These results suggest that the early diagnosis and comprehensive management make the history of alcoholism irrelevant as a prognostic factor in patients with cancer pain.

Current Status and Future Multidimensional Assessment

The present tools allow for the characterization of the intensity of different problems in palliative care patients. By rapidly assessing the intensity and different dimensions that are part of the given patient's problems, some of these tools can assist in the rapid development of a treatment strategy.

These tools are at different stages of development and may need further confirmation in prospective studies by other groups. Ideally, many of these assessments should be summarized in a tool package that will allow practitioners to obtain a rapid multidimensional assessment. This tool kit should also be available in simple software that might allow for recording the data for clinical purposes and also for quality control. Finally, the predictive accuracy of these different tools should be refined by incorporating new items or by improving the measurement of currently existing items. However, in the process of improving accuracy, it is crucial that the length of the overall assessments be kept short and that the effort for both patient and caregiver be kept to a minimum. Otherwise, these assessments will not be employed on regular care and they will not achieve their goal of improving the quality of palliative care in patients with advanced cancer.

OPIOID TOXICITY

During the past 15 years, the World Health Organization and numerous other organizations have emphasized the need for better assessment and management of cancer pain [1]. Opioids are now used not only in higher doses, but at earlier stages of the disease as compared to five to 10 years ago [18,19] as well as the adequate assessment and monitoring of cognitive and neuropsychiatric function in advanced patients [18-20].

This highly desirable increase in the use of opioids, combined with increased vigilance on neuropsychiatric status, has resulted in increased detection of several neuropsychiatric side effects.

In the following paragraphs, some of the literature characterizing key side effects and strategies for the management of these recognized toxicities will be reviewed.

Neuropsychiatric Side Effects

Table 2 summarizes the neuropsychiatric side effects of opioids. Most patients treated with opioid analgesics for the first time develop transient sedation or cognitive failure that resembles more the "slow-down" of cognition, rather than an increase in both numbers of errors or errors in judgment [21]. Delirium is frequent and under-diagnosed in patients with advanced cancer [13]. Opioids should be considered as a potential cause or as an aggravating factor in patients with delirium.

Table 2:   **Neuropsychiatric Side Effects**

- Cogntive failure
- Delirium
- Myoclonus/grand mal seizures
- hyperalgesia

Occasionally, patients receiving opioids may develop hallucinations with no cognitive failure [22]. These patients may be reluctant to describe their hallucinations for fear of being considered psychiatrically ill. In some cases a sudden change in the patient's mood (anxiety or depression) rather than obvious hallucinatory activity may indicate the development of organic hallucinosis.

Cases of myoclonus have been described after the administration of hydromorphone [23-25] meperidine [26,27], sufentanil and fentanyl [28]. Studies show that high concentrations of these opioids and their metabolites in cerebral spinal fluids (CSF) causes myoclonus [26].

Sjogren et al, described hyperalgesia and myoclonus that manifested both as generalized cutaneous hyperalgesia and progressive aggravation of cancer pain in patients receiving high doses of intravenous morphine [29]. These effects appeared to result from the accumulation of active opioid metabolites and responded to a switch in the opioid type [30,31].

Mechanism of Neuropsychiatric Toxicity

Animal studies have shown that morphine, morphine-3-glucuronide, normorphine, and hydromorphone are all capable of causing allodynia in rats after intrathecal high dosages [32-35]. Morphine, hydromorphone, and fentanyl are capable of causing agitation, myoclonus, hyperalgesia, and grand mal seizures in animals when administered systemically [34-38]. Evidence suggests that both tolerance and hyperalgesia share common neural substrates in the excitatory amino acids [33-37]. Animal evidence also suggests that some syndromes such as neuropathic pain combine the presence of hyperalgesia with decreased opioid responsiveness [35-38].

Animal and human studies have found that a variety of opioids including morphine, hydromorphone, and meperidine have active metabolites that are capable of causing significant neurotoxicity. These metabolites are generally produced in the liver and eliminated by urine. Conditions with increased circulating active metabolites include high opioid doses, prolonged treatment, dehydration, renal failure, and drugs that might decrease glomerular filtration. Some metabolites such as morphine-6-glucuronide are potent opioid agonists and therefore, are capable of causing the traditional opioid side effects including sedation and respiratory depression. Other metabolites such as morphine-3-glucuronide and normorphine are generally excitatory and do not bind to the opioid receptor. These metabolites are capable of causing agitation, myoclonus, hyperalgesia, and grand mal seizures. Because of the presence of mixed metabolites, most patients present with mixed syndromes combining sedation with excitation. In addition, a number of animal studies and clinical evidence suggest that parent compounds are also occasionally involved in severe neurotoxicity.

MANAGEMENT OF NEUROTOXICITY

If either the parent compound or its active metabolites are suspected to be at least partially responsible for neurotoxic toxicity, it would be reasonable to attempt an opioid rotation in order to decrease these side effects. A number of authors have reported significant improvement in neuropsychiatric side effects after opioid rotation [25-27,39,31,40]. The results should be interpreted cautiously because of the uncontrolled nature of the studies and the relatively small number of patients. However, in all cases the authors observed significant improvement after the opioid rotation. Most patients had severe symptoms of hyper-excitability. These results clearly justify randomized controlled trials on opioid rotation and suggest that opioid rotation should be tried in patients with acute neurotoxicity. The ideal alternative opioid has not been characterized. Initially, the trial of an alternative agonist such as hydromorphone or oxycodone is usually effective in patients who develop toxicity to morphine, and vice versa. In cases of severe toxicity after rotation among the most common opioid agonists, second line drugs such as methadone should be considered. Methadone has the advantages of extremely low cost, recently demonstrated NMDA antagonist properties and no active metabolites. However, its main disadvantages are a long and unpredictable half life and a poorly defined equianalgesic dose as compared to morphine and hydromorphone [40]. Methadone can be absorbed orally and rectally. It has a unique profile among other opioid agonists in that the equianalgesic dose appears to be relatively lower in patients previously exposed to high doses of opioid agonists as compared to patients previously exposed to low dosages [40]. These observations suggest that patients receiving other opioids develop only partial cross-tolerance to methadone. Randomized controlled trials on opioid rotation to methadone are currently being carried out. In the meantime, opioid rotation to methadone should only be performed by experienced specialists and such rotation should take place over several days in order to appropriately titrate the new opioid dose.

A number of reports suggest that dose reduction or discontinuation resulted in significant improvement in the patient's neuropsychiatric symptoms [39-41]. These observations further support the role of opioids as a cause for the patient's neurotoxic symptoms. However, both reduction or discontinuation are seldom possible in patients with advanced cancer.

Other measures including circadian modulation in order to titrate the dosing of opioid to the moments of maximal pain [42,43], hydration, in order to allow for a rapid elimination of active metabolites [44] and eventually the use of sedatives for patients who develop intractable excitatory side effects should also be considered [45]. The correct dose of opioid analgesics to control cancer pain is one that is effective and which is associated with manageable or acceptable toxicity. Unfortunately, the administration of opioids to opioid-naive patients can result in severe CNS side effects. In addition, a number of additional CNS adverse effects have been reported in patients treated with high doses of opioids over a long period of time. The prevention and adequate pharmacological treatment of such adverse effects is important to allow the ongoing treatment of cancer-related pain without sacrificing adequate analgesia.

Future studies are required to further the understanding of the role of opioid and non-opioid receptors, and the role played by the active metabolites of the different opioid analgesics in producing toxicity at the CNS level in cancer patients.

DEVELOPMENTS IN CANCER CACHEXIA

More than 80% of cancer patients will develop cachexia before death [46]. Cachexia is associated with a number of devastating symptoms, including anorexia, chronic nausea, asthenia, and changes in body image [46].

During recent years a number of effective symptomatic treatments have been developed for the management of some of these symptoms.

Pharmacological Interventions

Most cancers cause severe metabolic abnormalities, mainly characterized by profound lipolysis, decreased in skeletal muscle protein, and increased metabolic rate in addition to anorexia and decreased caloric intake [47]. Anorexia is seen more as a consequence of this central action of cytokines, tumor byproducts and the catabolic state due to the metabolic abnormalities, rather than as a cause of cachexia. Therefore, pharmacological interventions for cachexia can be aimed to the tumor, attempting to decrease the production of byproducts at the host immune system, attempting to decrease the production of cytokines by monocytes or to block the activity of these cytokines, or to the brain in order to prevent anorexia or stimulate appetite. In addition, recent research suggests that some pharmacological interventions could be directed at the muscles for the prevention or restoration of muscle mass and function.

Currently Available Drugs

Pro-kinetic agents: Autonomic failure with decreased gastric and intestinal motility is a recognized complication of cancer cachexia [48]. Metoclopramide and other pro-kinetic agents can improve these symptoms in patients with idiopathic, diabetic, and cancer-related autonomic failure [49]. Although very high doses have been used for chemotherapy-induced emesis [50] daily doses of 60-120 mg orally administered 4-6 hourly have been found to be effective. A recent randomized controlled trial has found that slow-release metoclopramide every 12 hours was significantly better than rapid-release metoclopramide every 6 hours, confirming the need for continued gastric stimulation for effective control of chronic nausea and early satiety [51]. The role of other pro-kinetic agents including domperidone and cisapride has not been established in randomized controlled trials in cancer patients.

Progestational Drugs: These drugs have been found to increase appetite, caloric intake, and improve weight in more than 10 randomized, controlled trials [46]. Both megestrol acetate and medroxyprogesterone acetate have been found to be effective. Recent studies have found that some of the subjective effects of progestational drugs do no result from weight gain, since patients with no significant change in nutritional status perceives significant symptomatic improvement [52,53]. Therefore, low dose megestrol acetate could result in symptomatic improvement without weight gain.

Corticosteroids: These drugs have an established role for the short-term symptomatic management of anorexia and chronic nausea in cancer patients [46]. They have no significant effect on nutritional status. However, they do have significant effects on pain and overall sensation of wellbeing. Because of their low cost and low toxicity, particularly when given for short periods, future clinical trials should attempt to compare corticosteroids with progestational drugs.

Emerging Drugs for the Management of Cachexia

Thalidomide: This drug has been found to inhibit tumor necrosis factor successfully in animal and human studies of leprosy, tuberculosis, cancer, AIDS and endotoxic injection [55-58]. In animals infected with endotoxin, thalidomide has been found to be able to significantly prolong survival [55]. In an open study on 30 patients with HIV infection and active tuberculosis, thalidomide was able to significantly reduce cytokine production. This was associated with significant improvement and accelerated weight gain. This drug is usually very well tolerated even in very symptomatic patients. Randomized clinical trials in cancer patients are justified. The fact that thalidomide has mild sedative effects might make the masking of these drugs in placebo controlled trials difficult.

Melatonin: This drug is able to decrease the level of circulating TNF in patients with advanced cancer [59]. It has also been found to be able to antagonize some of the side effects associated with the exogenous administration of TNF including asthenia and hypotension [60]. This drug is very well tolerated when administered orally. Therefore, randomized, placebo controlled trials in cancer cachexia should be conducted in order to better clarify its role.

Clenbuterol: This interesting drug belongs to a family of selective beta 2-adreno receptor agonists. It is closely related to the broncho dilator salbutamol and shares with such drugs some of the common side effects including nervousness, tachycardia, muscle tremors, and headache [61]. Clenbuterol has been found significantly increase muscle mass and function in exercising and sedentary rats. In addition, clenbuterol has been found to antagonize muscle protein waste in tumor-bearing rats [63]. One randomized controlled trial has found that clenbuterol was able to significantly improve muscle strength after knee surgery as compared to placebo [64]. This novel group of drugs with ability to prevent or reverse muscle loss even in sedentary populations which should be studied in randomized controlled trials against placebo.

In summary, after many years of minimal developments in the pharamcological management of cachexia, the last three years have seen a major resurgence of interest. Better definition of outcomes and a better understanding of the role of cytokines have assisted in the design of randomized clinical trials. A new and exciting series of compounds have proven in animal and initial human trials that it is justified to pursue randomized clinical trials.

REFERENCES

1. World Health Organization Expert Committee report 1990, Cancer pain relief and palliative care. Technical Series 804, Geneva, Switzerland: World Health Organization. pp 11-18.
2. Bruera E, MacDonald S. (1993) Audit Methods: The Edmonton Symptom Assessment System. In: I Higginson, ed, Clinical Audit in Palliative Care. Oxford: Radcliffe Medical Press 61-77.
3. Higginson I. (1993) Audit Methods: Validation and in-patient use. In: Higginson I, ed. Clinical Audit in Palliative Care. Oxford: Radcliffe Medical Press 48-54.
4. Fishman B, Pasternak S, Wallenstein SL, et al. (1987) The Memorial Pain Assessment Card. A valid instrument for the evaluation of cancer pain. Cancer 60:1151-58.
5. Portenoy RK, Thaler Ht, Kornblith AB, et al. (1994) The Memorial Symptom Assessment Scale. An instrument for the evaluation of symptom prevalence, characteristics and distress. Eur J Cancer 30A:1326-36.
6. Graham C, Bond SS, Genkovich MM, et al.(1980) Use of the McGill Pain Questionnaire in the assessment of cancer pain: replicability and consistency. Pain 8:377-87.
7. Dant RL, Cleeland CS, Flarery RC. (1983) Development of the Wisconsin Brief Pain Questionnaire to assess pain in cancer and other diseases. Pain 17:147-210.
8. de Haes JCJM, van Kipperberg FCE, Neijt JP. (1990) Measuring psychological and physical distress in cancer patients: structure and application of the Rotterdam Symptom Checklist. Br J Cancer 62:1034.
9. MCCorkle R, Young K. (1978) Development of a symptom distress scale. Cancer Nurs 1:373-78.
10. Au E, Loprinzi CL, Dhodapkar M, et al. (1994) Regular use of a verbal pain scale improves the understanding of oncology inpatient intensity. J Clin Oncol 12:2751-55.
11. Bruera E, Macmillan K, Hanson J, McDonald RN. (1989) The Edmonton staging system for cancer pain: preliminary report. Pain 37:203-209.
12. Bruera E, Schoeller T, Wenk R, MacEachern T, Marcelino S, Suarez-Almazor M, Hanson J. (1995) A prospective multi-center assessment of the Edmonton Staging System for cancer pain. J Pain & Symptom Manage 10(5):348-355.
13. Bruera E, Miller L, McCallion J, Macmillan K, Krefting L, Hanson J. (1992) Cognitive failure in patients with terminal cancer: a prospective study. J Pain Symptom Manage 7(4):192-195.
14. Smith MJ, Breitbart WS, Platt MM. (1995) A critique of instruments and methods to detect, diagnose, and rate delirium. J Pain Symptom Manage 10(1):37-77.
15. Pereira J, Hanson J, Bruera E. (1997) The frequency and clinical course of cognitive impairment in patients with terminal cancer. Cancer 79(4):835-42.
16. Breitbart W, Rosenfeld B, Roth A, Smith MJ, Cohen K, Passik S. (1997) The Memorial Delirium Assessment Scale. J Pain Symptom Mange 13:128-37.

17. Bruera E, Moyano J, Seifert L, Fainsinger RL, Hanson J, Suarez-Almazor M. (1995) The frequency of alcoholism among patients with pain due to terminal cancer. J Pain Symptom Manage 10(8):599-603.

18. Bruera E, Macmillan K, Hanson J, MacDonald RN. (1990) Palliative care in a cancer center: results in 1984 vs 1987. J Pain Symptom Manage 5(1):1-5.

19. Cancer Pain Release (1996). From Florianopolis (1994) to Santo Domingo (1996): A progress report on opioid availability. 9(1):4-5.

20. Breitbart W, Bruera E, Chochinov H, Lynch M. (1995) Neuropsychiatric syndromes and psychological symptoms in patients with advanced cancer. J Pain Symptom Manage 10(2):131-41.

21. Zacny JP, Lichtor JL, Thapar P, Coalson D, Flemming D, Thompson WK. (1994) Comparing the subjective, psychomotor and physiological effects of intravenous butorphanol and morphine in healthy volunteers. J Pharmacol Exp Ther 270(2):579-89.

22. Bruera E, Schoeller T, Montejo G. (1992) Organic hallucinosis in patients receiving high doses of opiates for cancer pain. Pain 48:397-399.

23. Eisele JH, Grigsby EJ, Dea G. (1992) Clonazepam treatment of myoclonic contractions associated with high-dose opioids: case report. Pain 49:231-2.

24. Babul N, Darke AC. (1993) Putative role of hydromorphone metabolites in myoclonus. Pain 52:123.

25. MacDonald N, Der L, Allan S, et al. (1993) Opioid hyperexcitability: the application of alternate opioid therapy. Pain 53:353-5.

26. Szeto HH, Inturrisi CE, Houde R, et al. (1977) Accumulation of normeperidine, an active metabolite of meperidine, in patients with renal failure or cancer. Ann Int Med 86:738-41.

27. Kaiko RF, Foley KM, Grabinski PY, et al. (1983) Central nervous system excitatory effects of meperidine in cancer patients. Ann Neurol 13:180-5.

28. Bowdle TA. (1987) Myoclonus following sufentanil without EEG Seizure Activity. Anesthes 67:593-5.

29. Sjogren P, Jonsson T, Jensen N-H, et al. (1993) Hyperalgesia and myoclonus in terminal cancer patients treated with continuous intravenous morphine. Pain 55:93-97.

30. Sjogren P, Jensen N-H, Jensen T-S. (1994) Disappearance of morphine-induced hyperalgesia after discontinuing or substituting morphine with other opioid agonists. Pain 59:313-3.

31. Sjogren P, Erikson J. (1994) Opioid toxicity. Current Opin Anesthesiol 7:465-69.

32. Woolf CJ. (1981) Intrathecal high dose morphine produces hyperalgesia in the rat. Brain Res 209:491-5.

33. Yaksh TL, Harty GJ, Onofrio BM. (1986) High dose of spinal morphine produce a nonopiate receptor-mediated hyperesthesia: clinical and theoretic implications. Anesthes 64:590-597.

34. Gong QL, Hedner J, Bjorkman R, Hedner T. (1992) Morphine-3-glucuronide may functionally antagonize morphine-6-glucuronide induced antinociception and ventilatory depression in the rat. Pain 48:249-55.

35. Mao J, Price DD, Mayer DJ. (1995) Mechanisms of hyperalgesia and morphine tolerance: a current view of their possible interactions. Pain 62:259-274.

36. Shohami E, Evron S.(1985) Intrathecal morphine induces myoclonic seizures in the rat. Acta Pharmacol et toxicol 56:50-54.

37. Mao J, Mayer DJ, Hayes RL, Price DD. (1993) Spatial patterns of increased spinal cord membrane-bound protein kinase C and their relation to increases in C-2-deoxyglucose metabolic activity in rats with painful peripheral mononeuropathy. J Neurophysiol 70:470-481.

38.   Ebert B, Andersen S, Krogsgaard-Larsen P. (1995) Ketobemidone, methadone and
       pethidine are non-competitive N-methyl-D-asparate (NMDA) antagonists in the rat cortex
       and spinal cord. Neuroscience Letters 187:165-168.

39.   de Stoutz ND, Tapper M, Fainsinger R. (1995) Reversible delirium in terminally ill
       patients. J Pain Symptom Manage 10:249-53.

40.   Bruera E, Pereira J, Watanabe S, Belzile M, Kuehn N, Hanson J. (1996) Opioid rotation
       in patients with cancer pain. A retrospective comparison of dose ratios between
       methadone, hydromorphone and morphine. Cancer 78(4):852-857.

41.   Caraceni A, Martini C, De Conno F, et al. (1994) Organic brain syndromes and opioid
       administration for cancer pain. J Pain Symptom Manage 9:527-33.

42.   Bruera E, Macmillan K, Kuehn N, Miller MJ. (1992) Circadian distribution of extra doses
       of narcotic analgesics in patients with cancer pain. A preliminary report. Pain 49:311-4.

43.   Bruera E, Fainsinger R, Spachynski K, Babul N, Harsanyi Z, Darke AC. (1995) Clinical
       efficacy and safety of a novel controlled release morphine suppository and subcutaneous
       morphine in cancer pain: a randomized evaluation. J Clin Oncol 13(6):1520-27.

44.   Fainsinger RL, MacEachern T, Miller MJ, et al. (1994) The use of hypodermoclysis for
       rehydration in terminally ill cancer patients. J Pain Symptom Manage 9:298-302.

45   Ripamonti C, Bruera E. (1997) CNS adverse effects of opioids in cancer patients.
       Guidelines for treatment. CNS Drugs 8(1):21-37.

46.   Bruera E, Fainsinger RL. (1993) Clinical management of cachexia and anorexia. In: D.
       Doyle, G. Hanks, N. MacDonald (Eds), Oxford Textbook of Palliative Medicine.
       London, England, Oxford Medical Publications, 4.3.6:330-37.

47.   Billingsly KG, Alexander HR. (1996) The pathophysiology of cachexia in advanced
       cancer and AIDS. In: Bruera E, Higginson I, eds. Cachexia-Anorexia in Cancer Patients.
       Oxford, Oxford University Press. 1:1-22.

48.   Bruera E, Catz Z, Hooper R, Lentle B, MacDonald RN. (1987)Chronic nausea and
       anorexia in patients with advanced cancer: a possible role for autonomic dysfunction. J
       Pain Symptom Manage 2(1):19-21.

49.   Pereira J, Bruera E. (1996) Chronic nausea. In: Bruera E, Higginson I, eds. Cachexia-
       Anorexia in Cancer Patients. Oxford: Oxford University Press 2:23-37.

50.   Gralla RJ, Itri LM, Pisko SE, et al. (1981) Antiemetic efficacy of high-dose
       metoclopramide: randomized trials with placebo and prochlorperazine in patients with
       chemotherapy-induced nausea and womiting. N Engl J Med 305:905-9.

51.   Bruera E, MacEachern T, Spachynski K, LeGatt D, MacDonald RN, Babul N, Harsanyi
       Z, et al (1994) Comparison of the efficacy, safety and pharmacokinetics of controlled
       release and immediate release metoclopramide for the management of chronic nausea in
       patients with advanced cancer. Cancer 74(12):3204-11.

52.   Bruera E, Ernst S, Hagen N, Spachynski K, Belzile M, Hanson J. (1996) Symptomatic
       effects of megestrol acetate (MA): a double-blind, crossover study. Proceed ASCO
       #1716; pg. 531.

53.   Tattersall MH. (1995) Tumor-related cachexia and the role of megestrol acetate
       (Abstract). 7th International Symposium on Supportive Care in Cancer, September 20-23,
       Eur J Cancer 12(2).

54.   De Conno F, Martini C, Caraceni A, et al. Megestrol acetate for anorexia in patients with
       advanced cancer. Personal communication - submitted for publication.

55.   Schmidt H, Rush B, Simonian G, et al. (1996) Thalidomide inhibits TNF response and
       increases survival following endotoxin injection in rats. J Surg Research 63(1):143-6.

56.   Schuler U, Ehninger G. (1995) Thalidomide: rationale for renewed use in immunological
       disorders (Review). Drug Safety 12(6):364-9.

57.   Tramontana JM, Utaipat U, Molloy A, et al. (1995) Thalidomide treatment reduces tumor necrosis factor alpha production and enhances weight gain in patients with pulmonary tuberculosis. Molecular Med 1(4):384-97.

58.   Kaplan G. (1994) Cytokine regulation of disease progression in leprosy and tuberculosis. Immunobiol 191(4-5):564-8.

59.   Lissoni P, Barni S, Tancini G. (1994) Role of the pineal gland in the control of macrophage functins and its possible implication in cancer: a study of interactions between tumor necrosis factor-alpha and the pineal hormone melatonin. J Biolog Regul & Homestatic Agents 8(4):126-9.

60.   Brackowski R, Zubelewicz B, Romanowski W, et al. (1994) Preliminary study on modulation of the biological effects of tumor necrosis factor-alpha in advanced cancer patients by the pineal hormone melatonin. J Biolog Regulat & Homeostatic Agents 8(3):77-80.

61.   Salleras L, Dominguez A, Mata E, et al. (1995) Epidemiologic study of an outbreak of clenbuterol poisoning in Catalonia, Spain. Public Health Reports 110(3):338-42.

62.   Rehfeldt C, Weikard R, Reichel K. (1994) The effect of the beta-adrenergic agonist clenbuterol on the growth of skeletal muscles of rats. Archiv fur Tierernahrung 45(4):333-44.

63.   Costelli P, Garcia-Martinez C,Llovera M, et al. (1995) Muscle protein waste in tumor-bearing rats is effectively antagonized by a beta 2-adrenergic agonist (clenbuterol). Role of the ATP ubiquitin-dependent proteolytic pathway. J Clin Investig 95(5):2367-72.

64.   Maltin CA, Delday MI, Watson JS, Heys SN, Nevison IM, Ritchie IK, et al. (1993) Clenbuterol, a beta-adrenoceptor agonist, increases relative muscle strength in orthopaedic patients. Clin Sci 84(6):651-4.

Multidisciplinary Approach to Pain Control

Fumikazu Takeda, M.D.

Neurosurgery Clinic, Saitama Cancer Center; WHO Collaborating Center for Cancer Pain Relief and Quality of Life, Ina, Saitama 362, Japan.

SUMMARY. Pain relief is a realistic target for the majority of cancer patients, so that health care workers should be appropriately educated about the updated knowledge and skills of pain management. Evaluation and treatment of cancer pain are best achieved by a team approach. The first steps are to take a detailed history, and to examine the patient carefully to determine the cause of the pain. Treatment should begin with an explanation and combined physical and psychological approach, using both drug and non-drug measures. Radiotherapy, nerve blocks and neurosurgical procedures are needed in a few cases. Nevertheless, analgesics and a limited number of other drugs are the mainstay of cancer pain management. Drugs are very effective when used along with the five key concepts: by mouth, by the ladder, for the individual, by the clock and attention to detail. National policy, teaching and training, opioid availability are the three important criteria in order to effectively implement a cancer pain relief programme in each country where cancer incidence and mortality are expected to continue to rise.

KEY WORDS: Cancer pain relief, Analgesic drugs, Policies, Education, Opioid availability

INTRODUCTION

Most persistent pains which include cancer pain must be controlled and, currently, can be controlled. Effective pain management is achieved when undertaken as part of comprehensive palliative care. Presently, however, many pains are treated inadequately. This is one of the main reasons why many health care workers continue to wrongly consider that most persistent pain is intractable. There is a widespread lack of awareness among them of the fact that effective approach exists to manage persistent cancer pain. In this paper, cancer pain relief, one of the most important international public health issues, is discussed according to the World Health Organization (WHO) strategies and guidelines [1] and author's clinical experience.

THE PRESENT GLOBAL STATUS

Incidence of pain in cancer

According to WHO [1], the number of cancer patients in the world is increasing. Of the estimated 9 million new cancer patients every year, more than half are in developing countries. Cancer incidence and mortality are expected to continue to rise in most regions of the world, mainly because of aging populations. Cancer patients need pain relief at all stages of their disease. Pain occurs in about one-third of patients receiving anti-cancer treatment. In these patients, pain relief measures and anti-cancer treatment should go hand in hand. In patients with advanced cancer, more than two-thirds experience pain, and the management of pain and other symptoms becomes the main realistic aim of the treatment. A conservative estimate is that every day globally at least 4 million people are suffering from cancer pain. Cancer pain is frequently managed inadequately even in the medically affluent areas of the world and is often not treated at all in many developing countries.

Reasons for inadequate relief

Since early 1980's, the WHO has summarized reasons why cancer pain is not adequately treated. They include the followings and seem to be also applicable when pain in non-malignant diseases is not adequately treated: 1) lack of awareness on the part of health care workers, health policy makers and administrators and the public that most cancer pain can be relieved; 2) limitation of health care delivery systems and personnel; 3) concern that medical use of opioid analgesics will produce psychological dependence and drug abuse. 4) legal restriction on the use and availability of opioid analgesics; and 5) absence of national policies on pain relief and palliative care.

WHO cancer pain relief programme

To respond to these issues, WHO launched a cancer pain relief programme in 1986. The objective of the WHO programme is to offer adequate pain relief to all cancer patients in the world through the existing health care systems. For effective programme implementation, WHO proposed three criteria. These are national policy, teaching and training, and opioid availability [1]. All three are interdependent with each other. Achievement in two areas without the third severely limits the programme implementation.

National policy: Establishment of a cancer pain relief and palliative care policy by national government should be a key priority in each country's health care system or as a part of its cancer control activities. A formulation of a policy that supports cancer pain relief through government endorsement of education and drug availability is central in the concerted effort to allow adequate pain relief. Australia, Canada, China, Japan, the Philippines, Sweden, USA, Vietnam and a number of other developed and developing countries recently established their national policies.

Teaching and training: Lack of systematic education in pain management has been existed in many countries. It is very encouraging to note, however, that an international close tie is developing between WHO, national

Table 1. Results of survey of Japanese nurses' knowledge in cancer pain management and continuing teaching and training (correct responses in % to questionnaires)

Groups Items	Nurses exposed to continuing education n=222	Nurses unexposed to continuing education n=141
Incidence of pain in cancer	70%	47%
The best judge of pain intensity	92%	77%
Use of placebo	64%	23%
Analgesics to be used	92%	59%
Route of administration	72%	34%
Indication of morphine	92%	53%
Reasons for increased doses	90%	69%
Psychological dependence	81%	19%

governments, leading medical societies, specialized centers and experts to make efforts in improving this common problem. More than several governments and leading medical societies have issued reports on cancer pain in recent years. There has been an increasing number of medical and nursing schools which have a teaching curriculum for pain relief and palliative care. Workshops and seminars on cancer pain relief and palliative care have been held in many areas of the world. For further improvement in the Western Pacific region, the WHO Regional Office plans to sponsor a regional workshop in Japan in March 1998. The title of the workshop will be "workshop in strengthening professional education in cancer pain relief and development of palliative care expertise".   Key experts and policy administrators representing 12 member states in the Western Pacific region will discuss in the workshop to effectively develop and implement their own national programmes.

In 1997, a survey conducted by a Japanese palliative care research group supported by the Ministry of Health and Welfare's New Ten Year Strategy Programme For Cancer Control definitely revealed an effect of continuing teaching and training. It shows a quite difference in knowledge level about cancer pain management between two groups of Japanese nurses: one which has been exposed to continuing teaching and training about WHO guidelines and another which has hardly been exposed to the continuing teaching and training. Table 1 shows percentage of correct responses from the respondents in each group to the questionnaires that asked them about incidence of pain in cancer, the best judge of pain intensity, use of placebo, analgesics to be used, indication of morphine, route of administration, reasons for increased doses and psychological dependence.

Opioid availability: Misunderstanding of tolerance and physical dependence and widespread undue fears of the dangers of psychological dependence are the major impediments to programme implementation. These have caused many doctors to use opioid analgesics in inadequate doses and sometimes to avoid their use altogether. However, neither tolerance nor physical dependence limits the doctor's ability to effectively use opioid analgesics, provided that the drugs are used correctly. Wide clinical experiences in many countries also demonstrated that psychological dependence does not occur in cancer patients receiving opioid analgesics for persistent pain. Recently, this was evidenced through animal experiments by Japanese pharmacologists [2]. Psychological dependence hardly occurred in the experimental animals receiving repeated administration of morphine and persistent pain stimulation, while it frequently occurred in those receiving repeated administration of morphine but not receiving the pain stimulation. It is suggested from the animal experiments that pharmacological activities induced in kapper-receptors by the pain stimulation participate to prevent psychological dependence. This information may help to avoid undue fears of the dangers of psychological dependence.

The United Nations International Narcotics Control Board (INCB) reported in 1995 special report that the need for opiates for legitimate medical purposes is not fully met, but the global annual consumption of morphine for medical purposes has been tripled in recent years due to increased use in pain relief [4] . Despite this increase, diversion of opioids from the licit trade into illicit channels remains relatively rare.

Morphine and other opioids are not available or available only under very strict conditions, because the national laws were established long before oral opioid analgesics became widely recognized as indispensable for effective treatment of cancer pain.   In such cases, it is essential for health care workers and drug regulators to cooperate in order to make opioid analgesics legally more available while preventing their abuse. It means that modification of laws and regulations to improve the availability of opioid analgesics is needed in many countries. Japan and the Philippines recently amended their pertinent national laws to improve the accessibility of opioid analgesics, notably morphine, to cancer patients for pain relief. Oral morphine preparations were legalized in India in 1987, in China in 1993 and in Vietnam in 1995 for the first time for national cancer pain relief programme implementation.

CAUSES AND NATURE OF PAIN IN CANCER

Appropriate clinical approach to pain needs comprehensive understanding of its causes and nature. Many patients with advanced cancer have multiple pains from several of the following categories: 1) Pain caused by cancer itself which is by far the most common. The cancer itself causes pain through extension into soft tissue, visceral involvement, bone metastases, nerve compression, nerve injury and raising intracranial pressure; 2) Pain related to cancer (e.g., lymphoedema, bedsore, etc.); 3) Pain related to anti-cancer treatment (e.g., chemotherapy-induced mucositis, etc.); and 4) Pain caused by a concurrent disorder (e.g., osteoarthritis, etc.).

Cancer pain is also classified according to its neural mechanism: 1) Nociceptive pain which is the most common and includes somatic, visceral and muscle spasm pain; 2) Neuropathic pain which includes nerve compression pain and nerve injury pain; and 3) Sympathetically-maintained pain.

Majority of cancer pain are persistent and usually becomes very severe in intensity as the disease advances. Severe persistent pain commonly causes fears and anxieties of the patient, interferes with the patient's quality of life and, thus, intensifies the patient's perception of the pain. The concept of total pain to encompass all relevant aspects is useful in cancer pain management. This includes the noxious physical stimulus and psychological, social and spiritual factors.

ASSESSMENT OF PAIN

Assessment or evaluation is a vital first step in adequate management of pain [1]. It is important for health care workers to believe the patient's report of pain. Pain is a purely subjective symptom, so that the health care workers should specifically ask the patient about pain, rather than relying on spontaneous comment. The severity of the pain should be evaluated by asking whether activity is limited by the pain, whether sleep is disturbed, and degree of relief obtained with past and present medication or pain-relief procedures.

A detailed history of the pain must be taken to discover the location and distribution of the pain, its quality and severity, whether it is continuous or intermittent, and what factors make it worse or better. It is important with a patient who under-report the severity of the pain and its impact on daily life to verify the history by speaking to a family member. The psychological state of the patient should also be evaluated. Information about past illness, concurrent level of anxiety and depression, and degree of functional incapacity help to identify patients who may require more specific psychological support. Detecting depression and other common psychiatric syndromes is an important part of the total evaluation.

A detailed history and a careful clinical examination may be all that is necessary to determine the cause of the pain so that appropriate treatment may begin. After initiating treatment, its results should be monitored continuously. Both continuing evaluation and treatment are best achieved by a team approach. The physician, nurse and other care-givers should regularly share information about the effects of treatment so that, when necessary, changes in treatment can be made quickly. The patients who feel and report the pain should also be considered as one of the team members.

TREATMENT STRATEGY

It is important to recognize that a sequence of specific aims is useful: increase of the hours of pain-free sleep; relief of the pain when at rest; and relief of the pain on standing or during activity. Treatment should begin with an explanation and combined physical and psychological approaches, using both drug and non-drug treatments. Radiotherapy may be useful to treat bone pain. Nerve blocks and neurosurgical procedures are supplementarily needed in a few cases. Anti-cancer treatment should concurrently carried out, if appropriate. Most pain responds well to a combination of a non-opioid and an opioid analgesics. With others which include bone pain and nerve compression pain, relief is obtained by combining a corticosteroid and an opioid. Neuropathic pains often show little response to non-opioid and opioid analgesics, but may be eased by the use of adjuvant drugs, namely, tricyclic antidepressants, anticonvulsants and local anesthetic congeners. Very anxious or deeply depressed patients may need an appropriate psychotropic drug in addition to an analgesic drug. If this fact is not appreciated, the pain often remains intractable.

Table 2.　A basic drug list for cancer pain relief*

Category	Basic drugs	Alternatives
Non-opioids	acetylsalicylic acid paracetamol ibuprofen indomethacin	choline magnesium trisalicylate diflunisal naproxen diclofenac
Opioids for mild to moderate pain 　(weak opioids)	codeine	dihydrocodeine dextropropoxyphene standardized opium tramadol
Opioids for moderate to severe pain 　(strong opioids)	morphine	methadone hydromorphone oxycodone levorphanol pethidine buprenorphine
Opioid antagonist	naloxone	
Antidepressants	amitriptyline	imipramine
Anticonvulsants	carbamazepine	valproic acid
Corticosteroids	prednisolone	prednisone

*Reproduced by permission of WHO, from Cancer Pain Relief, 2nd edition, Geneva, WHO, 1996 [1], Perm No. 97-265.

USE OF ANALGESICS

A limited number of drugs (Table 2) are needed to manage cancer pain, but they should be administered along with the five key concepts, namely, by mouth, by the ladder, for the individual, by the clock and attention to detail [1].

By mouth

Whenever possible, analgesics should be given by mouth.　In patients with dysphagia, uncontrolled vomiting or gastrointestinal obstruction, rectal suppositories and continuous subcutaneous infusion are useful alternative routes of administration.

By the clock

Analgesics should be given at fixed intervals of time. The next dose should be given before the effect of the previous one has worn off.　In this way, it is possible to relieve the pain continuously.

By the ladder

The sequential use of the drug according to the WHO three-step analgesic ladder is shown in Fig. 1. The first step is to use a non-opioid.　If a non-opioid does not relieve the pain, a weak opioid should be added. When a weak opioid in combination with a non-opioid fails to be effective, a strong opioid, notably morphine, should be substituted. Thus, if a drug ceases to be effective, a drug that is definitely stronger should be prescribed.

Morphine should be prescribed according to the intensity of the patient's pain, and not according to the brevity of prognosis.

For the individual

There are no standard doses for opioid drugs. The right dose is the dose that relieves the patient's pain for a length of time, preferably for four hours or more.   The range for oral morphine, for example, is from as little as 5mg to more than 1,000mg. Therefore, the initial dose should be 5 to 10mg every four hours and the dose should be titrated against the patient's pain, gradually increasing the dose until the patient is comfortable.

Attention to detail

It is essential to monitor the patient's response to the treatment to ensure that patient obtain maximum benefits with as few side-effects as possible. Such side-effects of an analgesics should be prevented by the concurrent use of adjuvant drugs which include anti-emetics and laxatives. The patient's psychological state should always be monitored, since psychological factors are the major influence to determine the intensity of the pain.

PROGRAMME IMPLEMENTATION IN JAPAN

The field-testing of the WHO method was carried out in Japan from 1982 to 1984 and evidenced the effectiveness and feasibility of the WHO method for relief of cancer pain for the first time in the world (Table 2) [3]. Further field-testing was carried out in several different countries with different health care systems. In each report, pain is completely relieved or considerably eased in the majority of cancer patients. Since 1989, Japan has had national policies for cancer pain relief, reinforced education of health care workers, and amended laws and regulations controlling narcotics. Workshops and seminars on cancer pain relief and palliative care have been held in many cities and areas, and a number of manuals, periodicals and monographs

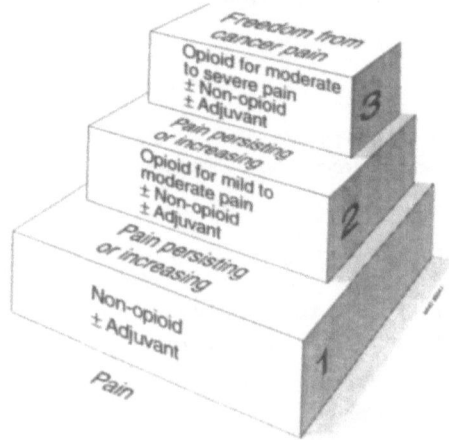

Fig.1. WHO Three-step analgesic ladder (Reproduced by permission of WHO, from Cancer Pain Relief, 2nd edition, Geneva, WHO, 1996 [1]. Perm No. 97-264)

Table 3. Results of field-testing in Japan of the WHO Draft Interim Guidelines for Relief of Cancer Pain (Saitama Cancer Center, 1985)

Analgesics	Step I Non-opioid (aspirin)	Step II Weak opioid (codeine)	Step III Strong opioid (morphine)	Ultimate result
No. of patients	86*	61**	118***	156
No. of patients with adjuvants	30	24	118****	
Complete pain relief	29 (33%)	29 (47%)	98 (83%)	136 (87%)
Acceptable pain relief	10 (12%)	12 (20%)	14 (12%)	14 (9%)
Partial pain relief	37 (43%)	15 (24%)	6 (5%)	6 (4%)
No pain relief	10 (12%)	5 (8%)	0	0

*Paracetamol was used in 6 patients.
**Paracetamol was concurrently used in 12 patients.
***Therapy was started on with morphine administration in 68 patients..
****Psychotropic drugs were used in 21patients.

have been published to educate health care workers. This year, the Ministry of Health and Welfare edited and distributed a cancer pain relief monograph in order to teach the public what can currently be done to effectively relieve cancer pain, since cancer pain relief is one of the priorities in cancer control programme in Japan.   Cancer has been the leading cause of death in Japan for the past 16 years.

As information dissemination has expanded nationwide with these efforts, annual morphine consumption for medical purposes has steadily increased in the past years.   It was 701kg in 1995, while it was 65kg in 1986. Nevertheless, the present annual consumption per capita is still much less than that in Canada, United Kingdom and United States. This fact reflects the cancer pain relief situation surveyed in 1996 by the ministry-sponsored palliative care research group. The survey result suggests that cancer pain management in Japan has much been improved as compared with that in some ten years ago, but nearly one-half of cancer pain patients are not satisfactorily relieved of their pain as yet.   Further effort should be made to disseminate information not only throughout Japan but globally that cancer patients have a right to demand and physicians a duty to administer sufficient doses of analgesics to control pain.

REFERENCES

1. World Health Organization (1996) Cancer Pain Relief. 2nd edition,WHO Publication Office, Geneva.
2. Suzuki T, Kishimoto Y, Misawa M (1996) Formalin- and Carrageenan-induced inflammation attenuates place preferences produced by morphine, methaphetamine and cocaine.   Life Sci   59: 1667-1674
3. Takeda F (1985) Results of field-tenting in Japan of the WHO Draft Interim Guideline on Relief of Cancer Pain. Pain Clinic 1:83-87
4. United Nations International Narcotics Control Board (1995) Availability of opiates for medical purposes. Report of International Narcotics Control Board for 1995. United Nations, New York

Malignant intestinal obstruction

Satoru Tsuneto[1], Masayuki Ikenaga[1], Jun Hosoi[1], and Tetsuo Kashiwagi[2]

[1]Hospice, Yodogawa Christian Hospital, 2-9-26 Awaji, Higashi-Yodogawa, Osaka 533, Japan
[2]Faculty of Human Sciences, Osaka University, 1-2 Yamada-oka, Suita, Osaka 533, Japan

SUMMARY. We conducted a prospective study of symptom prevalence in 206 terminally ill cancer patients and a retrospective study of the incidence and treatment of malignant intestinal obstruction in 110 patients (30 with gastric cancer, 30 with colon cancer, 30 with rectal cancer, and 20 with ovarian cancer). In the prospective study, pain was the most frequent symptom in patients surviving more than 1 month. The frequencies of general malaise, anorexia, constipation, and insomnia increased during the patient's final month. The frequency of confusion increased during the final 2 weeks. The frequencies of agitation and death rattle increased during the final days. The incidence of intestinal obstruction was 16%. In the retrospective study, we defined malignant intestinal obstruction as a final obstruction continuing for more than 1 week and for which surgery was not indicated. Malignant intestinal obstruction developed in 63% of patients with gastric cancer, 45% with ovarian cancer, and 40% with colorectal cancer. Symptoms of malignant intestinal obstruction in many patients were successfully controlled with opioids (morphine, buprenorphine, fentanyl), anticholinergic agents (scopolamine butylbromide, scopolamine hydrobromide), a major tranquilizer (haloperidol), and a somatostatin analogue (octreotide). Nausea and vomiting due to malignant intestinal obstruction were effectively treated in 75% of patients by continuous subcutaneous infusion of octreotide, with a median dose of 300 μg/day. However, a nasogastric tube was necessary in 33% of patients with ovarian cancer, 21% with gastric cancer, and 8% with colorectal cancer.

KEY WORDS: malignant intestinal obstruction, symptom prevalence, pharmacologic management, octreotide, nasogastric tube

INTRODUCTION

Malignant intestinal obstruction is a frequent complication of advanced or terminal abdominal and pelvic cancers. Surgery is the treatment of choice, but owing to the patient's poor general condition or advanced disease, surgery is appropriate for only a small percentage of patients. However, alternative management now available offers good symptom control. We studied symptom prevalence in terminally ill patients with gastric, colorectal, or ovarian cancers with special regard to the incidence and treatment of malignant intestinal obstruction.

METHODS

Our hospice, which is based in a hospital of 607 beds, can accommodate 23 patients. We conducted a prospective study of symptom prevalence in 206 terminally-ill cancer patients who died in our hospice from April 1993 through March 1994. We collected information on primary cancer sites, metastasis, symptoms, and survival.

We also performed a retrospective study with special regard to the incidence and treatment of malignant intestinal obstruction in patients with gastric, colorectal, or ovarian cancers. In this study we defined malignant intestinal obstruction as a final obstruction continuing for more than 1 week and for which surgery was not indicated. We reviewed the charts of 30 consecutive patients with gastric, colon, or rectal cancers and of 20 consecutive patients with ovarian cancers who died in our hospice from February 1994 through July 1997. We collected the following information: incidence of malignant intestinal obstruction; symptoms of malignant intestinal obstruction such as pain, nausea, and vomiting; and the effectiveness of treatment.

RESULTS

Demographics of Terminally Ill Cancer Patients

Two hundred six patients (100 men and 106 women) who had been admitted to our hospice from April 1993 through March 1994 were enrolled in the prospective study (Table 1).

Table 1. Demographics of terminally ill cancer patients

No. of patients	206
Gender (male/female)	100 / 106
Age (years)	62.5 ± 12.9
Hospice stay (days)	28.8 ± 29.9

The distribution of primary cancer sites in our hospice population was similar to that in patients dying of cancer throughout Japan (Table 2). Stomach cancer was the most common, followed by lung cancer, colon/rectum cancer, breast cancer, and liver cancer. About half of these patients had metastases to the lung, and others had metastasis to the peritoneum, liver, bone, or brain (Table 3).

Table 2. Primary cancer site (n=206)

Stomach	19%
Lung	17%
Colon · rectum	14%
Breast	10%
Liver	7%
Pancreas	5%
Uterus	5%
Biliary tract	5%
Others	17%

Table 3. Metastasis (n=206)

Lung	48%
Peritoneum	46%
Liver	40%
Bone	28%
Brain	12%

Symptom Prevalence

We investigated the cumulative frequency of symptoms in the 206 patients and considered symptoms to be present even when controlled with treatment. The three most prevalent symptoms were malaise, anorexia, and pain (Table 4).

Table 4. Symptom prevalence until death (n=206)

General malaise	98%
Anorexia	95%
Pain	77%
Constipation	75%
Insomnia	63%
Dyspnea	52%
Nausea · vomiting	46%
Confusion	32%
Death rattle	25%
Ascites	24%
Pleural effusion	24%
Intestinal obstruction	16%

Symptom Prevalence and Length of Survival

Figure 1 shows the relationship between the main symptoms and the length of survival in the 206 patients. The length of survival was defined as the period from the onset of symptoms until death. Pain was the most frequent symptom when the length of survival was more than 1 month. The frequencies of general malaise, anorexia, constipation, and insomnia increased during the final month. The frequency of confusion increased during the final 2 weeks. The frequency of agitation and death rattle increased during the final days.

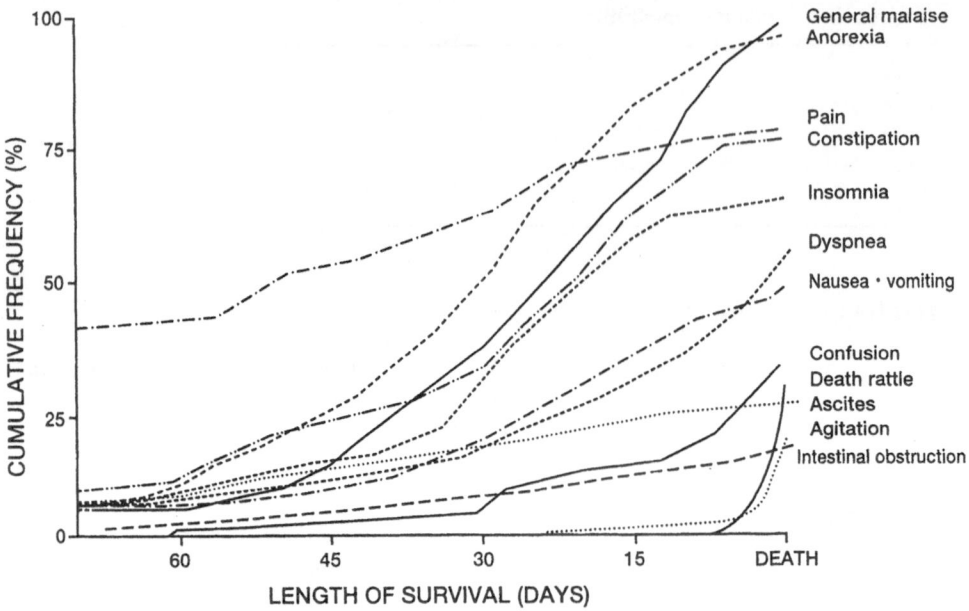

Figure 1. Length of survival from the onset of symptoms

Demographics of Patients with Gastric, Colon, Rectal and Ovarian Cancers

Table 5 shows the demographics of patients with gastric, colon, rectal and ovarian cancers who died in our hospice from February 1994 through July 1997 and were investigated by our retrospective study. Gastric and ovarian cancers metastasized to the peritoneum and caused ascites much more often than did colorectal cancers. In contrast, colorectal cancer metastasized to the liver much more often than did gastric and ovarian cancers.

Table 5. Demographics of patients with gastric, colon, rectal and ovarian cancers

Primary cancer	No.	Peritoneal metastasis (%)	Ascites (%)	Liver metastasis (%)
Stomach	30	77	40	23
Colon	30	37	23	63
Rectum	30	17	17	50
Ovary	20	75	55	20

Malignant Intestinal Obstruction and Length of Survival

Malignant intestinal obstruction developed in 63% of patients with gastric cancer, 45% of patients with ovarian cancer, and 40% of patients with colorectal cancer (Table 6).

Table 6. Incidence and length of survival of malignant intestinal obstruction (n=110)

Primary cancer	No.	Obstruction (%)	Median survival (day)
Stomach	30	63	30
Colon	30	40	29
Rectum	30	40	25.5
Ovary	20	45	22

Pain due to Malignant Intestinal Obstruction

Patients experienced both continuous pain and colic pain due to malignant intestinal obstruction. In each type of cancer, continuous pain was more common than colic pain (Table 7).

Table 7. Pain due to malignant intestinal obstruction (n=52)

Primary cancer	No.	Continuous pain (%)	Colic pain (%)	Effectiveness of treatment (%)
Stomach	19	58	36	85
Colon	12	67	50	82
Rectum	12	25	25	100
Ovary	9	44	33	67

Continuous pain was treated with three opioids: morphine, buprenorphine, and fentanyl (Table 8). These opioids were usually infused subcutaneously, except for buprenorphine, which was administered sublingually. Colic pain was treated with intravenous and continuous subcutaneous infusion of butylbromide scopolamine.

Table 8. Pharmacological management of pain due to malignant intestinal obstruction

Medication	No.	Median dose (range) mg/day	Route of administration
Morphine	8	44 (10 - 180)	CSI
Buprenorphine	8	0.55 (0.2 - 1.68)	CSI
	4	0.6 (0.4 - 1.6)	SL
Fentanyl	3	0.72 (0.6 - 0.85)	CSI
Scopolamine butylbromide	4	40 (40 - 60)	IV
	3	96 (50 - 200)	CSI

CSI : Continuous subcutaneous infusion
SL : Sublingually

Nausea and Vomiting due to Malignant Intestinal Obstruction

Nausea and vomiting were more frequent in patients with gastric or ovarian cancer than in patients with colorectal cancer (Table 9). A nasogastric tube was more often necessary in patients with ovarian or gastric cancer.

Table 9. Nausea and vomiting of malignant intestinal obstruction (n=52)

Primary cancer	No.	Nausea and vomiting (%)	Nasogastric tube(%)	Effectiveness of treatment (%)
Stomach	19	84	21	75
Colon	12	67	8	75
Rectum	12	58	8	100
Ovary	9	100	33	67

Nausea and vomiting due to malignant intestinal obstruction was treated with haloperidol, metoclopramide, scopolamine hydrobromide, and scopolamine butylbromide (Table 10). In most cases these agents were continuously infused subcutaneously, except for metoclopramide, which was administered intravenously.

Table 10. Pharmacological management of nausea and vomiting due to malignant intestinal obstruction

Medication	No.	Median dose (range) mg/day	Route of administration
Haloperidol	21	10 (4-20)	CSI
Metoclopramide	25	40 (20-100)	IV
	3	100	CSI
Scopolamine hydrobromide	6	0.75 (0.5-3.0)	CSI
Scopolamine butylbromide	4	73 (40-200)	CSI

CSI : Continuous subcutaneous infusion

Malignant intestinal obstruction was treated with continuous subcutaneous infusion of octreotide (Table 11). No side effects were observed.

Table 11. Treatment of malignant intestinal obstruction by continuous subcutaneous infusion of octreotide (n=22)

Median dose (μ g/day)	300 (120-600)
Median duration (day)	14 (1-62)
Effectiveness (%)	75

DISCUSSION

Previous studies have reported that malignant intestinal obstruction occurs in 3% to 15% of terminally ill cancer patients [1,2]. Our prospective study found that malignant intestinal obstruction developed in 16% of cancer patients who died in our hospice. This high incidence is probably due to the high rate of gastric cancer in the general population and to careful observation at the time of death. Colorectal, gastric, ovarian, and uterine cancers are most commonly associated with malignant intestinal obstruction [3,4]. The reported incidence range of malignant intestinal obstruction is 5.5% to 42% in ovarian cancer and 10% to 28% in colorectal cancer [5-7]. We found that malignant intestinal obstruction developed in 63% of patients with gastric cancer, 45% with ovarian cancer, and 40% with colorectal cancer.

Surgical treatment should be considered for every patient with intestinal obstruction. Reported survival rates after palliative surgery for malignant intestinal obstruction range from 2.5 to 11 months [3-5]. Chan and Woodruff reported a morbidity of 80% and a postoperative (within 30 days) mortality of 40% among 10 patients with malignant intestinal obstruction who were treated surgically [8]. Surgery is considered to have been beneficial if the patient survives for at least 2 months [3,5]. However, owing to the patient's poor general condition or to advanced disease, surgery is indicated for only a small percentage of these patients.

In our retrospective study, we defined malignant intestinal obstruction as a final obstruction continuing for more than 1 week and for which surgery was not indicated. The median survival of our patients with malignant intestinal obstruction was less than 1 month. However, reported survival times after the onset of malignant intestinal obstruction vary widely. Baines and colleagues reported a mean survival of 3.7 months [1]. Isbister and colleagues reported that their patients survived 29.2 days [9]. These differences in survival are probably due to differences in definition, assessment, determination, surgical intervention, and time of diagnosis.

In many patients with gastric, colon, rectal, or ovarian cancers the symptoms of malignant intestinal obstruction were successfully controlled with opioids (morphine, buprenorphine, fentanyl), anticholinergic agents (scopolamine butylbromide, scopolamine hydrobromide), and a major tranquilizer (haloperidol). However, a nasogastric tube was necessary in 33% of patients with ovarian cancer, 21% with gastric cancer, and 8% with colorectal cancer.

Octreotide is a relatively new agent for treating nausea and vomiting [10,11]. Octreotide is a long-acting somatostatin analogue which reduces intestinal secretion and suppresses the release of intestinal peptide hormones. Seventy-five percent of our patients with malignant intestinal obstruction responded to continuous subcutaneous infusion of octreotide, with a median dose of 300 μ g/day and a median duration of 14 days. This response rate is comparable to those of previous reports [10,11]. However, a nasogastric tube was necessary in some patients with malignant intestinal obstruction.

In conclusion, these findings suggest that malignant intestinal obstruction in many terminally ill cancer patients can be treated pharmacologically with minimal use of a nasogastric tube.

REFERENCES

1. Baines M, Oliver DJ, Carter RL (1985) Medical management of intestinal obstruction in patients with advanced malignant disease. Lancet 2 : 990-993
2. Fainsinger R, Spachynski K, Hanson J, Bruera E (1994) Symptom control in terminally ill patients with malignant bowel obstruction. J Pain Sympt Manage 9(1) : 12-18
3. Mercadante S (1997) Assessment and Management of Mechanical Bowel Obstruction. In : Portenoy RK, Bruera E (eds). Topics in Palliative Care. Oxford University Press, New York, pp 113-130
4. Baines M (1997) The pathophysiology and management of malignant intestinal obstruction. In : Doyle D, Hanks GWC, MacDonald N (eds). Oxford Textbook of Palliative Medicine. 2nd ed. Oxford University Press, Oxford, pp 526-534
5. Ripamonti C (1994) Management of bowel obstruction in advanced cancer patients. J Pain Symptom Manage 9(3) : 193-200
6. Frank C (1997) Medical management of intestinal obstruction in terminal care. Can Fam Physician 43 : 259-265
7. Waller A, Caroline NL (1996) Handbook of Palliative Care in Cancer. Butterworth-Heinemann, Boston, pp 181-188
8. Chan A, Woodruff RK (1992) Intestinal obstruction in patients with widespread intraabdominal malignancy. J Pain Symptom Manage 7(6) : 339-342
9. Isbister WH, Elder P, Symons L (1990) Non-operative management of malignant intestinal obstruction. JR Coll Surg Edinb 35 : 369-372
10. Khoo D, Hall E, Motson R, Riley J, Denman K (1994) Palliation of intestinal obstruction using octreotide. Eur J Cancer 30A(1) : 28-30
11. Mangili G, Franchi M, Mariani A, Zanaboni F, Rabaiotti E, Frigerion L, Bolis PF, Ferrari A (1995) Octreotide in the management of bowel obstruction in terminal ovarian cancer. Gynecol Oncol 61 : 345-348

Session Summary

Symptom Control in Palliative Medicine: Standard Management and Clinical Trials I

Kenji Eguchi[1], Jean Klastersky[2]

[1] National Shikoku Cancer Center, Matsuyama, Japan
[2] Institut Jules Bordet, Bruxelles, Belgium

At the opening of this session, Prof. Jean Klastersky made some brief comments on the importance of symptom control and quality of life research in patients with incurable diseases. He pointed out several obstacles to research in this area including the poor sensitivity of measurements, the lack of appropriate methods to analyze information censoring, and multiplicity data. Further efforts will be necessary to find ways to deal with these problems and achieve a breakthrough in symptom control for patients with incurable diseases.

The session began with a presentation by Prof. Eduardo Bruera, who focused on pain research and cachexia. Many reports have shown a discrepancy between doctors and patients in the perceived severity of symptoms. He mentioned various instruments for measuring symptoms, such as ESAS and a new staging system for cancer pain. These instruments are available without copyright through the Internet (http.//www.palliative.org). He then discussed various mechanisms of opioid toxicity and strategies for opioid management, such as methadone and opioid rotation. Although several small pilot studies of cancer cachexia and anorexia have been performed, extensive research is still required to clarify etiology, mechanisms, and treatment. Answering questions regarding the pathogenic mechanisms of tumor necrosis factor (TNF) in cancer cachexia and trials on the feasibility of an anti-TNF antibody, he stated that more scientific studies are needed to clarify the multiple mechanisms of cachexia/anorexia syndrome in cancer patients. Thus far, the effectiveness of combinations of anti-TNF antibodies and other drugs have not been confirmed in clinical trials.

In response to a question on the relationship between zinc deficiency and asthenia-depression-anorexia syndrome, Prof. Bruera answered that two small pilot studies of oral zinc administration conducted in the United Kingdom in the mid-1980's failed to show a definitive correlation between hair zinc content and the severity of symptoms. He added, however, that current methods of zinc measurement are unreliable. As a general comment, the role of cancer centers has become more important to educate and commit the level of palliative medicine in the community. Oncologists at cancer centers should share innovative knowledge bt collaborating with researchers in academic medicine.

The second speaker, Prof. Fumikazu Takeda, presented his views, as a member of the World Health Organization (WHO) Pain Relief Program Committee, on the current status of pain management according to the WHO Pain Relief Program. He reviewed the history of the development of the ladder scheme for analgesia use established by the Committee in the early 1980's. He stressed five aspects of analgesic treatment to which medical staff should pay attention: by mouth, by the clock, by the ladder, for the individual, and attention to detail. Continuing education for personnel involved in palliative medicine is also important to achieve better pain control. Concerning the deletion of the second step in the WHO three-step ladder strategy, he said that the strategy was proposed in the early 1980's when morphine was not legally available in all countries. Currently, he said, morphine is readily available for medical purposes and that the two-step ladder can easily be modified for bedside practice. Education for patients and lay people was also important to decrease misunderstanding and the fear of opioid dependence. He mentioned that dependence did not develop when opioids were used for pain control in an experimental animal model. In response to a question, Dr. Takeda said that pharmacokinetic and pharmacodynamic studies support the appropriate use of opioids in palliative medicine.

The third talk, by Dr. Satoru Tsunetou, a hospice physician at Yodogawa Christian Hospital, Osaka, focused on the management of malignant intestinal obstruction. He outlined hospice activities and reported that a high percentage of patients with terminal gastric, colorectal, or ovarian cancer suffer from intestinal obstruction. He presented his experience with such treatments as insertion of nasogastric tubes, palliative surgery, and octreotide. He reported that the indications for palliative surgery were a single site of obstruction, life expectancy more than 2 months, good performance status, and informed consent. Octreotide costs $150 to $200 per day and is indicated as a second-line treatment after other drugs, such as scopolamine, have failed. Several members of the audience commented on the need for a structured algorithm based on scientifically evaluated data for the management of malignant intestinal obstruction including, for example, indications for nasogastric tube placement and the efficacy and limitations of octreotide.

Prof. Klastersky closed this session with his comment that clinical research is needed on symptom control in palliative medicine. Multicenter collaborative studies of each topic are warranted to replace anecdotal evidence at single institutions. Subcommittee activities of the Multinational Association for Supportive Care in Cancer such as pain, nausea, and vomiting, are progressing in the same direction as the goals stated above.

Session II

Symptom Control in Palliative Medicine: Standard Management and Clinical Trials II

Chairpersons:
Geert H. Blijham and Fumikazu Takeda

The Treatment of Chronic Nausea in Patients with Advanced Cancer

Ronald Feld, MD

FRCPC, FACP, The Princess Margaret Hospital, University of Toronto, Toronto, Ontario Canada

Summary. Chronic nausea with no apparent cause lasting longer than one month occurs in most patients with advanced malignancy, especially in those patients admitted to palliative care units just prior to death. Unfortunately this syndrome has been poorly studied to date, compared to other types of nausea and vomiting, particularly that associated with cytotoxic chemotherapy. Autonomic dysfunction possibly associated with opioid and non steroidal anti-inflammatory drug use is the likely cause. Aggressive approaches to this type of nausea can control the symptom complex in most patients. The combination of metoclopramide plus corticosteroids is the backbone of therapy. Early data suggests that 5HT3 antagonists may also be beneficial in this syndrome but prospective randomized controlled trials are required to confirm this. Research on this subject is the only way to make progress and further improve the quality of life of patients with advanced malignancy, especially in the time just prior to their death.

Key Words: Nausea, Vomiting, Chronic, Malignancy, Palliative

Much has been written about the treatment of nausea and vomiting in cancer patients during the 1980s and 1990s due to the rapid advances made in new therapy for this serious side effect of chemotherapy, which frequently interferes with compliance [1,2,3]. In contrast very little has been written about emesis associated with the terminal cancer patient. This syndrome includes nausea, vomiting and can also include anorexia. Chronic nausea is a frequent symptom in these patients with a prevalence frequently involving a third of patients and in some series up to just under 70% of such patients [4,5,6,7]. Vomiting in these patients is probably less commonly seen (about 30% of patients). It has been defined in some studies as lasting at least one month associated with advanced malignancy with all other potential causes ruled out [8]. It has also been noted that patients with stomach and breast cancer have higher rates of nausea and vomiting than other patients with terminal malignancies [4].

Reuben et al in a paper published in 1983, [4] reported on just under 1600 patients terminally ill from the National Hospice Study. In this study nausea and vomiting occurred in 62% of patients with 30% of patients found to have this symptom in the final 6 weeks of their life. Another study by Dunlop looked at patients' perception of gastrointestinal symptoms and weakness [9]. Fifty patients ranked the relative frequency and distress of a number of gastrointestinal symptoms. Nausea was the 8th most frequent symptom and vomiting the 10th. Dry retching appeared as the 20th most frequent and 22nd most distressing symptom. Females ranked this symptom higher than males [9].

Andrews and Hawthorne have studies emesis in animals and have divided it up into pre-ejection, ejection and post ejection phases [10]. That many stimuli cause emesis suggests that several pathways may be involved. A review of the various theories is beyond the scope of this manuscript but some new perspectives on this topic have recently been reviewed [2]. Suggestions of new avenues to explore include substance P. antagonists [11,12] and perhaps octreotide [13]. Great advances have also been made in the neuropharmacology of emesis. The discovery of a variety of neurotransmitters, many of which can be blocked by classical antiemetics has been well studied in animals. This has been confirmed in man primarily by the fact that antiemetics thought to block specific pathways seem to be quite effective.

The general principles governing the treatment of chronic nausea and vomiting in this patient population are very important. In patients with chronic nausea, the general environment of the patient, body odours, diet, quality and amount of food and it's presentation must all be seriously considered. Also a good knowledge of pharmacological principles related to nausea and vomiting are necessary [14]. Single agent antiemetic therapy can be tried but frequently combinations are used in which each agent acts by a different mechanism. The agents used in the past for all types of nausea in cancer patients were primarily phenothiazines (example:prochlorperazine) and butyrophenones (example:haloperidol) but more recently 5HT3 receptor antagonists usually combined with corticosteroids have become very popular. The latter have been particularly useful for very severe emesis associated with combination chemotherapy in cancer patients, particularly cisplatin based [1,2]. Benzodiazepines, particularly short acting ones, also seem to be useful and probably work on the limbic system [14]. The control of nausea and vomiting by psychological technics can be effective but is frequently time consuming. Acupuncture has shown some promise against cytotoxic induced emesis but may also be useful in other settings [14]

In the case of chronic nausea and vomiting in patients with advanced cancer, it becomes essential to rule out other common causes of nausea and vomiting of which there are many [14,15]. As detailed in Table I, some of the potential causes in this patient population include poor hygiene of the oral and nasopharynx, fungating growths in the head and neck region, oesophageal obstruction due to intrinsic or extrinsic tumors. Gastric stasis can occur in variety of settings including the presence of hepatomegaly or ascites, as well peptic ulcers and pancreatic cancer and can cause vomiting. Certainly bowel obstruction can also be a serious problem particularly in patients with gynaecological or other intra-abdominal malignancies.

Table 1. Causes of nausea and vomiting in patients with advanced malignancy

Gastro intestinal	Metabolic
Head & neck (fungating growths)	Hypercalcaemia
Herpes simplex	Uraemia
Esophageal Obstruction	Ketosis
Gastric stasis	"Toxins"
Peptic ulcer	
Gastritis	Drugs
Bowel obstruction	Opioids
Pancreatitis	Digoxin
	NSAID
Central Nervous system	Chemotherapy
CNS cancer 1^0 or 2^0	Other
Meningitis	Chronic Nausea
Vestibular disturbances	
	Radiation
	Abdominal or pelvic
	Brain

Another potential cause is cerebral or other intracranial metastases. Metabolic causes also are potential reasons for chronic nausea. These include uraemia, hypercalcemia and occasionally ketosis, often associated with diabetes mellitus or just from severe vomiting. Among the most frequent causes of nausea in this population is the concomitant use of opioids [6,16] and or non steroidal anti-inflammatory agents, frequently used for pain relief in this population [12]. The nausea and vomiting associated with opioids often dissipates after several days of therapy but can sometimes continue to cause the symptom complex. Obviously cytotoxic chemotherapy can cause emesis but at the time of the terminal phase of their disease patients with malignancy are usually not given cytotoxic agents. On the other hand they may be given radiation therapy for the relief of other symptoms which may in turn contribute to nausea.

Chronic nausea is often associated with anorexia and weight loss and can arise from all the etiologies previously mentioned. Bruera and colleagues from Edmonton suggest that it may be most frequently associated with opioid treatment and/or autonomic dysfunction [8].. In order to make this diagnosis one has to rule out all the other potential causes previously mentioned, usually with investigations but they should at least be ruled out on a clinical basis. As previously mentioned, at least in the study setting this syndrome has been defined as nausea lasting more than one month, having eliminated the many other causes previously described [8].

Gastroparesis has been studied as a cause of this syndrome in the past but a recent study by Nelson and colleagues from the Cleveland clinic [17] was particularly interesting. They investigated 30 patients, 10 with no malignancy and early satiety, 10 with malignancy and no early satiety and normal volunteers without malignancy. They evaluated them looking at gastrointestinal motility and also administered a questionnaire. Patients with early satiety, particularly those with reduced motility had more abnormal answers on their questionnaires. The authors were concerned that because their control arm of volunteers were considerably younger than the study subjects, this could have been a source of bias. They used a simple test with markers which were 1 cm sections of nasogastric tubing in which a radio-opaque line was embedded. This was well tolerated and seemed to identify the abnormalities of gastric motility quite easily. The authors recommended this should be used more generally to identify gastroparesis. Because of their findings, they also recommended that treating these patients with metoclopramide or other prokinetic agents might be the treatment of choice.

Bruera and colleagues from Edmonton Alberta, among the most frequent authors on the subject of chronic nausea, felt that the most important cause of the problem in this population was dysfunction of the autonomic nervous system as noted in one of their studies [18]. It was manifested by impaired gastric emptying and abnormal cardiovascular autonomic tests. They determined the former by using a gastric emptying scan. They gave all 5 patients on study an egg sandwich labelled with 99 TC Sulphur Colloid. The point at which half of this sandwich was consumed was designated as time 0. Sequential counts were recorded with the patients standing up every 10 minutes for 90 minutes. Blood pressure measurements and ECGs were also carried out. Bruera found that abnormal gastric emptying was the prime cause of nausea and anorexia in their patients in their pioneering study. This kind of problem has also been seen in diabetics [19] and in lung [20] and pancreatic cancer patients [21]. Bruera concluded that the presence of delayed gastric emptying in their study justified a clinical trial to study anti-dopaminergic drugs (e.g. metoclopramide) or cholinergics (e.g. betanechol) which have both demonstrated an effect on gastric emptying time.

In 1994 Bruera and his colleagues published a manuscript in which 29 evaluable patients were included [8]. In this study patients were randomized in a double blind crossover design to receive 40 mg of metoclopramide by continuous infusion every 12 hours or 20 mg of immediate release metoclopramide every 6 hours. The nausea intensity was measured (after each treatment) using both a categoric scale and visual analogue scale (VAS) as recommended by others [22]. The VAS scores for nausea for the three treatment days of study were significantly lower for patients who received the controlled release metoclopramide compared to those who received the immediate release metoclopramide (p=0.047). However, using the categoric scale, nausea scores were not significantly different between treatments taking into account the time of day and days across the three treatment days. The authors concluded that controlled release metoclopramide is safe and effective in managing chronic nausea in patients with advanced cancer. In addition to their clinical observations, the authors noted there were also excellent blood levels sustained with the controlled release agent. This reduced the need for more frequent dosing. Also little or no toxicity was observed with this treatment. Obviously serious limitations for using this kind of medication occurs in patients who are unable to swallow intact tablets, since crushing of tablets may result in a bolus drug effect. They recommended that future studies should focus on better characterization of the syndrome and that they should more clearly determine the optimum dose of metoclopramide. As well they suggested studying the effects of drug combinations such as those already proven useful at the time of publication in managing chemotherapy induced emesis (that is metoclopramide plus corticosteroid). At the time of their study 5HT3 receptor antagonists were not readily available.

Bruera and colleagues recently published a retrospective review of 100 consecutive patients admitted to the palliative care unit at the Edmonton General Hospital during the period 1992 to 1993 [23]. Interestingly prior to death, virtually all the patients developed chronic nausea. They initially treated patients who complained of nausea with metoclopramide 10 mg every 4 hours orally or subcutaneously. If nausea persisted for more than 2 days, dexamethasone 10 mg twice a day was added. After 2 days if this don't work, they then used a continuous subcutaneous infusion of metoclopramide in a dose of 60 to 120 mg per day plus dexamethasone in the same dose as before.
If still no response was observed or further or toxicity prevented the use of the antiemetics chosen after 2 days, other antiemetics were administered. These included drugs such as haloperidol, dimenhydrinate and cisapride which were used sequentially. Their conclusion was that although nausea is frequent, it can be well controlled in the majority of patients using safe and simple antiemetic regimens. Following their steps, as outlined above, other agents were infrequently required. Of interest is a recent retrospective study suggesting the benefit to using ondansetron in a variety of patients with debilitating diseases including a small number of patients with advanced malignancy [24]. Megastrol acetate has also been noted to be of some benefit in this syndrome [25].

Although chronic nausea in advanced cancer is a frequent and very debilitating problem, research on the subject has been lacking. Research should be strongly encouraged but reasonable approaches for treatment of this syndrome are already available as described and should be utilized to keep these patients as comfortable as possible in the last days of their life. We hope to soon see the results of completed research on some of the newer antiemetic agents alone or in combination with older agents and to see if they offer any additional benefits over those already established to be beneficial.

REFERENCES:

1. Warr D. Standard treatment of chemotherapy induced emesis. Supportive Care in Cancer 1997;5:12-16.
2. Herrstedt J. New perspectives in antiemetic treatment. Supportive Care in Cancer 1996;4:416-19.
3. Hesketh PJ. Treatment of chemotherapy induced emesis in the 1990's: Impact of the 5HT3 receptor antagonists. Supportive Care in Caner 1994;2:286-92.
4. Reuben DB, Mor V. Nausea and vomiting in terminal cancer patients. Arch Intern Med

1983;146:2021-3.

5. Faisinger R, Bruera E, Miller MJ, Hanson J, MacEachern T.   Symptom control during the last week of life on a palliative care unit.   J Palliat Care 1991;7:5-11.

6. Curtis EB, Krech R, Walsh TD.   Common symptoms in patients with advanced cancer.   J Palliat Care 1991;7:25-9.

7. Blaines M.   Nausea and vomiting in patients with advanced cancer.   J Pain Symptom Manage 1988;3:81-5.

8. Bruera Ed, MacEachern TJ, Spachynski KA, LeGatt DF. MacDonald RN, Babul N, Harsanyi Z, Darke AC.   Comparison of the efficacy, safety and pharmacokinetics of controlled release and immediate release of metoclopramide for the management of chronic nausea in patients with advanced cancer.   Cancer 1994;74:3204-11.

9. Dunlop GM.   A study of the relative frequency and importance of gastrointestinal symptoms and weakness in patients with far advanced cancer. Palliative Medicine 1989;4:37-43.

10. Andrews PLR and Hawthorn J.   The neurophysiology of vomiting.   Ballieres Clinical Gastroenterology 1988;21:141-68.

11. Andrews PLR.   the mechanism of emesis induced by chemotherapy and radiotherapy.   IN antiemetics in the supportive care of patients.   Ed. M. Tonato ESO Monograph, Springer Verlag Berlin, Germany 1996 pp.3-24.

12. Andrews PLR and David CJ.   The physiology of emesis induced by anticancer therapy.   In: Serotonin and scientific basis of anti-emetic therapy.   Eds J Reynolds, PLR Andrews and CJ Davis - Oxford Clinical Communication, Oxford UK, 1995;25-49.

13. Mosdell KW, Visconti JA.   Emerging indications for octreotide therapy.   I, II AM. J. Hosp Pharmacy 1994;5:1184-1192 and 1318-1330.

14. Allan SG.   Nausea and vomiting.   In: Oxford Textbook of Palliative Medicine Eds.   Doyle D Hanks GWC and MacDonald, Oxford University Press, Oxford England 1993, pp 282-90.

15. Lichter I.   Results of antiemetic management in terminal illness.   J Palliat Care 1993;9:19-21.

16. Walsh TD, West TS.   Controlling symptoms in advanced cancer.   BMJ 1988;296:477-81.

17. Nelson KA, Walsh TD, Shechan FG, O'Donovan PB, Falk GW.   Assessment of upper gastrointestinal motility in the cancer associated dyspepsia syndrome.   J Palliat Care 1993;9:27-31.

18. Bruera ED, Catz Z, Hooper R, Lentle B, MacDonald RN.   Chronic nausea and anorexia in advanced cancer patients: A possible role for autonomic dysfunction.   J Pain Symptom Manage 1987;2:19-21.

19. Ewing D, Campbell I, Clarke B.   Assessment of cardiovascular effects in diabetic autonomic neuropathy and prognostic implications.   Ann Int Med 1980;92-308-11.

20. Schuffler M, Wallace H, Fleming C, Bell CE, Bouldin TW, Malagelada JR, McGill DB, LeBauer SM, Abrams, Love J.   Intestinal pseudo-obstruction as the presenting manifestation of small-cell carcinoma of the lung: A paraneoplastic neuropathy of the gastrointestinal tract.   Ann Int Med 1983;98:129-34.

21. Barkin JS, Goldberg RI, Sfakianakis GN, Lei J.   Pancreatic carcinoma is associated with delayed gastric emptying.   Digestive Diseases & Science 1986;31:265-7.

22. Morrow GR.   The assessment of nausea and vomiting - Past problems, current issues and suggestions for future research.   Cancer 1984;53:2267-78.

23. Bruera E, Seifert L, Watanabe S, Babul N, Darke A. Harsanyi Z, Suarez-Almazor M.   Chronic nausea in advanced cancer patients: A retrospective assessment of a metoclopramide-based antiemetic regimen.   J Pain Symptom Manage 1996;11:147-53.

24. Currow DC, Couglan M, Fardell B, Cooney NJ.   Use of ondansetron in palliative medicine.   J Pain symptom Manage 1997;13:302-7.

25. Loprinzi CL, et al.   Controlled trial of megastrol acetate for the treatment of cancer, anorexia and cachexia.   J N.C.I.   1990;82:1127-32.

THERAPY OF FEBRILE NEUTROPENIA : AN ALGORITHM FOR CURRENT CLINICAL ATTITUDES TAKING INTO ACCOUNT COST BENEFIT

Jean KLASTERSKY[1]

[1] Professor and Chief of Medicine; Service de Médecine et Laboratoire de Recherche et d'Investigation Cliniques H.J. Tagnon, Institut Jules Bordet, Centre des Tumeurs de l'Université Libre de Bruxelles, Bruxelles, Rue Héger-Bordet 1, 1000 Bruxelles, Belgique

The treatment of febrile neutropenia has changed over the past 20 years and still is in a constant phase of reevaluation in relationship to modifications of the nature of the offending pathogens, availability of new drugs for treatment of infections and changes in the type of patients who become neutropenic as a consequence of cytostatic therapy (1).

The present review will deal with recommendations for the treatment of febrile neutropenia, with a special attention to its cost benefit. Cost-effectiveness evaluation is difficult and can be influenced by many biaises. Our conclusions will be based on the daily expenses for medical care of febrile neutropenia in Belgium (expressed in US dollars) as they are presently charged to the social security services (Table 1).

Table 1
Daily cost of various interventions for the management of febrile neutropenia

	Belgian francs	US dollars	Yens
Hospital stay	12 966	350	38 900
Day care clinic	6 562	177	19 680
At home nurse's visit	516	14	1540
At home doctor's visit	587	16	1 760
Ceftazidime (6g)	3 759	101	11 270
Meropenem (3 g)	3 423	92	10 260
Ceftriaxone (4 g)	2 598	70	7 790
Amikacin (1.5 g)	1 407	38	4 220
Vancomycin (2 g)	2 948	80	8 840
Amoxicillin/clavulanate (1875 mg)	264	7	790
Ciprofloxacine (1500 mg)	228	6	680
Filgrastim (300 µg)	4 176	113	12 530
Amphotericin B (75 mg)	408	11	1240

Monotherapy versus combination therapy

Two decades ago, when the main problem during febrile neutropenia was Gram negative bacillary bacteremia, combination therapy with a beta-lactam plus an aminoglycoside was standard. The IATCG (International Antimicrobial Therapy Cooperative Group) used successfully the combination ceftazidime/amikacin as the standard combination therapy and actually demonstrated that, in patients with severe protracted neutropenia and documented Gram negative bacillary bacteremia, a full course of amikacin with ceftazidime was superior to ceftazidime supplemented by only a limited number of amikacin administrations (2).

However, Gram negative bacteremia has become less frequent and new broad specrum agents have appeared, making monotherapy an appealing approach to avoid the toxicity of aminoglycosides. The IATCG has compared meropenem to ceftazidime/amikacin and found both treatments similarly effective as empiric therapy of febrile neutropenia (3). Not only the initial response rates were similar but mortality, further infections, addition of a glycopeptide or of an antifungal agent were not different, as summarized in Table 2.

In terms of expenses, meropenem costs 92 US dollars daily and ceftazidime/amikacin 139; other expenses for these therapies, which are both given 3 times daily, are probably very similar in hospitalized patients. Freifeld et al. compared monotherapy with ceftazidime to imipenem and found a similar efficacy in terms of initial response and subsequent complications (4). The respective daily dosage was for 90 mg/kg for ceftazidime and 50 mg/kg for imipenem leading to an average daily cost of 101 and 92 US dollars respectively.

Elting et al. found that patients with Gram negative bacillary bacteremia had a similar outcome whether treated initially with monotherapy or combination; however those patients who received the combination stayed on therapy for a mean duration of 7.2 days while those receiving monotherapy stayed for 8.9 days (5). As indicated in Table 3, if we calculate the cost for ceftazidime/amikacin and meropenem, the benefit in terms of cost of drugs is 1001-819=182 US dollars in favor of monotherapy. Assuming that the patients were discharged by the end of antibiotic treatment, the respective costs for hospital stay were 2520 and 3115 US dollars respectively with a 595 US dollars advantage for the combination. Thus overall, there might be a cost advantage for the combination, in spite of the lower cost of monotherapy, because of the reduced duration of the hospital stay. Moreover, in patients with proven Gram negative bacteremia, combination therapy is more active than monotherapy especially in patients with prolonged and severe granulocytopenia (2). Since Gram negative bacteremia represents only 7 % of the febrile neutropenic episodes today, the aminoglycoside can be discontinued early in most patients started on combination therapy in whom no bacteremia will be demonstrated.

Table 2
Meropenem vs Ceftazidime + Amikacin

	Meropenem n = 483		Ceftazidime + Amikacin n = 475	
Response				
Overall	270/483	(56 %)	245/475	(52 %)
Microbiologically documented	54/125	(43 %)	41/129	(32 %)
Bacteremia	47/113	(42 %)	34/114	(30 %)
Clinically documented	61/126	(66 %)	145/226	(64 %)
Mortality at day 30 :				
Overall	24	(5 %)	22	(5 %)
Related to infection	8	(2 %)	13	(3 %)
Further infections :				
Overall	56	(12 %)	58	(12 %)
Bacteremias	12	(2 %)	13	(3 %)
Addition				
Glycopeptide	160	(33 %)	182	(38 %)
Antifungal agent	112	(23 %)	119	(25 %)

IATCG-EORTC & GIMEMA, 1996

Table 3
Cost (in US dollars) of a treatment of febrile neutropenia
with monotherapy or combination therapy

	Monotherapy	Combination therapy
Duration of therapy (days)	8.9	7.2
Cost of antibiotics*	92 x 8.9 = 819	139 x 7.2 = 1001
Cost of hospitalisation	350 x 8.9 = 3115	350 x 7.2 = 2520
Total costs	3934	3521

*meropenem vs ceftazidime/amikacin

Coverage of Gram positive infections

As already mentionned, there has been a considerable change in the nature of the pathogens involved in febrile neutropenia (Table 4). Presently, most bacteremias during episodes of febrile neutropenia are caused by coagulase-negative staphylococci, which are usually resistant to methicillin, and by various strains of streptococci that are not always fully sensitive to penicillins, penems and third generation cephalosporins. It has been proposed therefore to include glycopeptides (vancomycin or teicoplanin) in the empiric regimens to be used in febrile neutropenic patients to cover for penicillin or methicillin resistant organisms.

The IATCG conducted a randomized study comparing ceftazidime/amikacin to ceftazidime/amikacin/vancomycin (6). Gram positive bacteremia responded more often in the vancomycin arm (72 % vs 43 %, p = 0.01), i.e. modifications of protocol antibiotic therapy occurred less often and much later in patient treated with ceftazidime/amikacin/vancomycin. However, the proportion of febrile patients at each treatment day in the 2 treatment regimens was not different and the mortality rate for patients with Gram positive bacteremia was 1 % for ceftazidime/amikacin arm and 3 % for the other arm. Table 5 indicates the modifications of empiric therapy that occurred in the 2 study groups. Antibiotics were changed in 50 % of the patients receiving empirically ceftazidime/amikacin and in 42 % in the other group. Vancomycin was usually added in the patients treated with ceftazidime/amikacin. However, antifungals were given significantly more often to the patients who had received vancomycin from the start. The addition of antiviral drugs and other antibiotics was not different in the 2 study groups.

Table 4
Bacteremias in EORTIC-IATCG trials

	I (1973-78)	II (1978-80)	III. (1980-83)	IV (1983-86)	V (1986-88)	VIII (1989-91)	IX (1992-94)
Bacteremias/ febrile episodes (%)	145/453 (32)	115/419 (27)	141/582 (24)	219/872 (25)	213/749 (28)	151/694 (22)	161/706 (22)
Gram negative (%)	103 (71)	74 (64)	85 (59)	129 (59)	78 (37)	47 (31)	53 (33)
E.coli	46	33	38	63	45	20	22
P.aeruginosa	18	18	23	34	14	10	10
Gram positive (%)	42 (29)	37 (36)	58 (41)	90 (41)	135 (63)	104 (69)	108 (67)
S.aureus	28	10	14	26	20	13	10
S.coagulase-negative	5	9	24	21	49	39	53
S.pneumoniae	5	6	4	6	0	3	0
Other streptococci	0	0	14	35	46	45	40
Other Gram positives	4	12	2	3	16	4	5

Table 5
Modification of antimicrobial therapy in the overall study population

	Ceftazidime + Amikacin	Ceftazidime + Amikacin + Vancomycin	
No. patients	370	377	
Any antimicrobial agent	184 (50)	158 (42)	.04
Antibiotics	118 (32)	44 (12)	<.001
Vancomycin	81	0	
Other	37	44	
Antifungals	44 (12)	86 (23)	<.001
Amphotericin B	38	81	
Acyclovir	30 (8)	43 (11)	.16

IATCG-EORTC & the National Cancer Institute of Canada, 1991

From the cost-benefit point of view, there might be an advantage for the ceftazidime/amikacin arm compared to the other regimen, since vancomycin costs 80 US dollars daily. However, as mentionned above, 81 patients out of 370 received vancomycin following initial therapy with ceftazidime/amikacin and 38 received amphotericin B in that group. In the other group, no patient received vancomycin and 81 patients received amphotericin B. As therapy was maintained for 10 days in most of the patients in both groups, and changes were made usually on the third day for vancomycin and on day 5 for amphotericin B, one can calculate the cost of therapy in the 2 arms of the the IATCG study (Table 6). It can be seen that treating Gram positive infections with glycopeptides only when these infections are microbiologically documented is highly cost-effective.

Table 6
Cost of the IATCG study of ceftazidime/amikacin (370 patients)
versus ceftazidime/amikacin/vancomycin (377 patients) in US dollars

	Ceftazidime/Amikacin	Ceftazidime/Amikacin /Vancomycin
Vancomycin empirical (10 days)	——	800 x 377 = 301 600
Vancomycin added (7 days)	560 x 81 = 45 360	——
Amphotericin added (5 days)	55 x 38 = 2 090	55 x 81 = 4 455
Total	47 450	306 055

In an other study, Elting et al. (5), in 909 episodes of bacteremia, did not demonstrate either an increased mortality when patients with Gram positive infections received delayed vancomycin therapy; however, that strategy increased the duration of therapy by 25 % (11.8 days vs 8.6 days; p = 0.01). If one translates these observations to our model, postulating that vancomycin is added on day 3, after unsuccessful empiric therapy without vancomycin, and that patients are discharged by the end of therapy, the cost of therapy with or without initial therapy with vancomycin for patients with Gram positive bacteremia can be estimated as indicated in Table 7. It can be seen that the costs are somewhat lower when vancomycin is given initially in patients wit bacteremia; in the other patients vancomycin is added later (usually on day 3) and a full therapy (± 7 days) with that agent explains the increased cost due to extended hospital stay. However Gram positive bacteremia represents only 15 % of the febrile episodes; as discussed earlier, the very high cost of vancomcyin does not justify its use in all patients with febrile neutropenia for a modest cost benefit (864 dollars per patient) in only 15%. Actually, the empiric addition of glycopeptides in non responding patients to initial therapy is probably not justified unless a resistant Gram positive microorganisms has been isolated (7). The IATCG is presently studying that question in a prospective randomized blinded trial.

Table 7
Cost in US dollars and per patient of initial or delayed therapy with
vancomycin in patients with gram positive bacteremia*

	No initial vancomycin	Initial vancomycin
Duration of therapy (days)	11.8	8.6
Cost of vancomycin**	688	944
Cost of hospital stay	4 130	3 010
Total Cost	4 818	3 954

* Gram positive bacteremia represents 15 % of the febrile neutropenic episodes
** Given from the onset or added on day 3

Out patient therapy of febrile neutropenia

Talcott et al. have proposed to separate patients with febrile neutropenia in different prognostic categories (8). Their work is being successfully validated by the MASCC (Multinational Association for Supportive Care in Cancer) subcommittee for infections. It is clear that the patients, with controlled neoplastic disease, without serious non neoplastic co-morbidity and who are not hospitalized at the time of the febrile neutropenic episode, do not present any serious morbidity and have a minimal mortality during or after the episode. These patients are good candidates for out patient therapy.

Outpatient therapy can consist of intravenously administered drugs or orally given antibiotics. For intravenous administration, at home or in the clinic, a once a day regimen would be particularly appealing. The IATCG compared the efficacy and toxicity of single daily ceftriaxone/amikacin and multiple daily doses of ceftazidime/amikacin (9). The single daily dosing of ceftriaxone/amikacin was as effective and not more toxic than multiple dosing of ceftazidime/amikacin. Oral therapy with amoxicillin-clavulanate/ciprofloxacin has been found comparable in efficacy to various intravenous regimens (10). A comparison between amoxicillin-clavulanate/ciprofloxacin and ceftriaxone/amikacin is now conducted by the IATCG; no difference in efficacy or toxicity could be detected so far.

As indicated in Table 8, oral antibiotics, even with the added cost of daily close surveillance by a physician and a nurse, have an optimal cost-benefit. If intravenous administration is desirable, using a once a day regimen, substantial savings can still be achieved by having the patient visited daily the out patient clinic or by having therapy given and supervised at home.

Table 8
Total cost per day (in US dollars) of 2 regimens suitable for
out patient therapy of febrile neutropenia

	Ceftazidime + amikacin	Ceftriaxone + amikacin	Amoxicillin/ clavulanate + ciprofloxacin
In hospital	489	458	363
Daily visit to clinic	—	285	190
At home*	—	148	43

* daily visited by physician and nurse

Hematopoietic growth factors

Randomized trials of granulopoietic growth stimulating factors in febrile patients with neutropenia have not consistently shown clinical benefit. A recent study assigned randomly 138 patients to receive G-CSF or a placebo in afebrile outpatients with severe chemotherapy induced neutropenia (11). The median time to an absolute neutrophil count > 500 x cu mm was significantly shorter for patients who received G-CSF (2 days versus 4 days). However, there was no effect on the rate of hospitalization, numbers of days in the hospital, duration of treatment with parenteral antibiotics or number of culture positive infections.

A meta-analysis of older studies by Messori et al. (12) shows that, in patients with small cell lung cancer, G-CSF did not affect mortality but significantly reduced the incidence of neutropenic fever (Table 9). That pharmaco-economic analysis, to estimate the cost-effectiveness ratio of preemptive G-CSF, found however that this cost-effectiveness profile was not particularly favorable (14 372 US dollars to prevent of one episode of febrile neutropenia).

Table 9
Study-specific rates of fever with neutropenia and
mortality and results of the meta-analysis

	Cumulative rate of fever with neutropenia over 6 cycles		Mortality rate from infection	
	G-CSF	Control	G-CSF	Control
First author				
Crawford	38/954	80/1044	3/957	3/1017
Trillet-Lenoir	12/655	31/645	1/655	3/645
Wolls	22/341	22/341	4/341	1/341
Pooled rates*	38.7 %	68.3 %	3.9 %	3.5 %
Relative risk of				
fever or death	0.29 P<0.001	1	1.13 P=0.82	1

* from Crawford et al., Trillet-Lenoir et al., Wolls et al.

Adapted from Messori et al.

As an adjunct to induction chemotherapy for adult acute lymphoblastic leukemia, G-CSF reduced dramatically the duration of neutropenia; the median time to reach levels of neutrophils > 500 x cu mm was 16 days with G-CSF versus 26 days; it significantly reduced the incidence of febrile neutropenia (12 % versus 42 %) and documented infections (40 % versus 77 %) (13). The overall survival was unchanged. It is possible that a cost benefit of prophylactic G-CSF would be more clearcut in patients with more severe and prolonged neutropenia; however, in this study the duration of hospitalization was not stated and the cost-effectiveness of G-CSF was just speculated upon as the authors felt that « a potential reduction in the number of hospital stays due to accelerated neutropoietic reconstitution by G-CSF may also translate into a socioeconomic benefit ». However, in patients with acute leukemia, many other factors than the duration of granulocytopenia may cause prolongation of the hospital stay.

In established febrile neutropenia, a recent randomized trial in pediatric patients (14) showed that patients randomized to G-CSF had a shorter hospital stay (5 versus 7 days) and fewer days on antibiotics (5 versus 6 days) resulting in a modest cost saving in treating neutropenic sepsis (1035 US dollars per patient). In another study, Maher et al. also demonstrated a cost saving for therapy with G-CSF of febrile neutropenia (15); the benefit was related to a reduction of severe (< 500 x cu mm) neutropenia which translated into a reduced hospital stay (5 versus 8 days).

These 2 studies, summarized in Table 10, indicate a cost benefit for the patients who received G-CSF at the same time as empirical antibiotics for the treatment of febrile neutropenia. This advantage is clearly related to the significant reduction of the duration of hospitalization. The results for GM-CSF are shown in Table 11; Maher's study favors GM-CSF but Vellenga's is negative. Anaissie's study has not evaluated costs but differences in clinical outcome do not appear significant (16, 17). As discussed by Schimpff (18), it should be stressed that neither study included patients at the greatest risk of complications, i.e. those with prolonged and severe neutropenia, as those with acute myelocytic leukemia or allogeneic marrow or stem cell transplantation.

Table 10
Effect of addition of G-CSF to antibiotics for the
treatment of febrile neutropenia (median values)

	Maher (1993)		Mitchell (1997)	
	G-CSF	Placebo	G-CSF	Placebo
Neutrophil recovery < 500 (days)	1*	6*	3*	5*
Hospital stay (days)	5*	8*	5*	7*
Febrile days	1	2	2	3
Days on antibiotics	5	5	5*	6*
Cost (US dollars)	3 600	5 900	4 147	5 169

* statistically significant

Table 11
Effect of addition of GM-CSF to antibiotics for the
treatment of febrile neutropenia (median values)

	Maher (1993)		Vellenga (1996)		Anaissie (1996)	
	GM-CSF	Placebo	GM-CSF	Placebo	GM-CSF	Placebo
Neutrophil recovery	1*	6	3	3	7	8
Hospital stay (days)	5*	8	6	7	9	10
Febrile days	2	2	4	4	4	4
Days of antibiotics	5	5	5	5	7	8
Cost (US dollars)	3600	5900	4100	500	-	-

* statistically significant

Prophylaxis of bacterial infections

A recent meta-analysis of studies using prophylaxis with fluoroquinolones in neutropenic patients indicate that fluoroquinolones alone are effective in preventing Gram negative bacteremia, and that a combination of fluoroquinolones plus penicillin, vancomycin or macrolides significantly reduced the occurrence of Gram positive bacteremia (19). Fever-related morbidity had an overall odd ratio of 0.76 for quinolones alone and 0.83 for quinolones plus anti-Gram positive coverage. In other words, the use of prophylaxis avoids 20 % of the episodes of febrile neutropenia, especially those leading to bacteremia.

Based on the figures used in this review (Table 3 and Table 7), a single episode of febrile neutropenia costs approximately 4600 US dollars. On the other hand, the frequency of febrile neutropenia in chemotherapy-treated patients is highly variable depending on the type of chemotherapy administered; intensive or standard chemotherapy were found associated respectively with a 48 % and a 11 % incidence of febrile neutropenia (20).

At the Institut Bordet, we perform each month about 15 high dose treatments and 300 standard dose treatments. The potential consequence of a systematic use of prophylaxis among our patients is indicated in Table 12. It appears that prophylaxis is cost effective in patients who are treated with high dose chemotherapy in whom the risk of neutropenia in the range of 50 %, but not in patients with standard dose chemotherapy who have a lower risk of febrile neutropenia.

Table 12
Expected savings from prophylaxis (amoxicillin/clavulanate plus ciprofloxacin) in patients treated with chemotherapy*

	High dose chemotherapy	Standard dose chemotherapy
Number of therapy courses	15	300
Number of febrile neutropenias°	7 (45%)	30 (10 %)
No. of avoided episodes by prophylaxis (20 %)°°	1.5	6
Cost of prophylaxis (US dollars)	2925**	31 200***
Cost of prevented episodes°°°	6 900	27 600
Net gain	3 975	-3 600

* monthly, at the Institut Jules Bordet, ** all patients for 15 days, *** all patients for 8 days
° Blay et al., °° Cruciani et al., °°° Cost of one episode : 4600 US dollars

Discussion

Febrile neutropenia is a changing syndrome which requires periodical updates as our therapeutical armementarium and techniques evolve. Changes in the microbial flora responsible of infections in neutropenic patients occur as well and new patterns of resistance appear, under the pressure of antibiotic use. In addition, cost of therapy has become a major issue when designing therapeutic strategies to be used in large number of patients.

Because of its high mortality in the 60's, due mainly to Gram negative bacillary infections, febrile neutropenia was considered as an oncological emergency to be treated with combinations of antibiotics in a hospital environment. However, since these early days (1), Gram negative bacillary bacteremia has become less frequent and has been replaced by more indolent Gram positive coccal infections. It is likely, although unproven, that these changes were influenced by the use of prophylactic antibiotics in neutropenic patients.

Moreover it became clear that all neutropenic are not alike (8); Talcott's observation that, among patients with febrile neutropenia, a group with minimal morbidity could be detected has been validated by the MASCC subcommittee for infections. It has been shown also that short-lived febrile neutropenia - today the most common presentation - can be adequately managed in an outpatient setting (10). It is therefore important to develop predictive models of the severity and duration of neutropenia like that presented by Blay et al. (20). Finally, the availability of the hematopoietic growth factors allows to reduce significantly the duration of neutropenia and potentially translate into clinical benefit.

At the present time, the mortality due to the infection itself, during an episode of febrile neutropenia is in the range of 2 %; in addition to that, further infection and progressive cancer explains the overall 10 % mortality in patients with febrile neutropenia (21). Most patients, especially if neutropenia is of short duration, have an uneventful course once treated with antibiotics; about 50 % become afebrile 3-4 days after the onset of therapy and in the others, it is common to have modifications of the initial treatment made at that time, which ensure eventually a favorable outcome. The usual duration of hospitalization is 7-8 days and the average cost, under these circumstances, is in the range of 4600 US dollars.

There is a trend towards monotherapy for the treatment of febrile neutropenia (22); third generation cephalosporins and penems are preferred to the classical combination therapy including beta-lactams and aminoglycosides. However, if one takes into account that combination therapy is associated with a shorter stay of bacteremic patients in the hospital (5), which reduces the cost, and also leads to a better response rate in those patients with Gram negative bacillary bacteremia and prolonged severe neutropenia (2), it might be wise to recommend initial combination therapy for febrile episodes in patients whose neutropenia is expected to last for more than 10 days. In these patients, if Gram negative bacillary bacteremia is not documented or if the duration of neutropenia is actually shorter than expected, combination therapy is no longer needed and can be discontinued early, avoiding potential problems associated with prolonged administration of aminoglycosides.

However, Gram negative bacillary sepsis is presently found in about 5 % of the patients with febrile neutropenia. It may be asked whether it is advisable to prescribe aminoglycosides to all patients for the benefit of only few. However, using the Talcott's criteria (8) and predictive rules for prolonged neutropenia (20), one should be able to limit the prescription of combination therapy to relatively small numbers of patients at high risk. As already mentionned, aminoglycosides can be safely discontinued after 48/78 hours if blood cultures do not confirm the presumptive diagnosis of Gram negative bacillary bacteremia or if granulocytopenia subsides.

Empiric prescription of a glycopeptide is not only useless, provided some coverage of streptococcal infections is given, but definitely very expensive. Clearly, the addition of a glycopeptide to the initial empiric therapy, only when it is dictated by the isolation of a microorganism specifically sensitive to it, is effective (7). The observation that patients with Gram positive bacteremia who receive a glycopeptide from the onset of therapy stay less longer in the hospital and thus cost less, cannot justify the systematic use of glycopeptides for empiric therapy. Gram positive bacteremia represents only 15 % of the episodes of febrile neutropenia seen today and, moreover, the emergence of vancomycin-resistant enterococci and staphylococci, that has been linked to an excess of prescription glycopeptides and cephalosporins, represent a major threat.

The demonstration by Talcott et al. (8) that among the population of febrile neutropenic patients existed a subgroup with a better prognosis in terms of morbidity and mortality opened the way for ambulatory therapy of febrile neutropenia (10). This subgroup represents about 25 % of patients with febrile neutropenia.

As indicated in Table 8, out patient treatment either in a day care facility (285 US dollars) or under close supervision at home (148 US dollars) with ceftriaxone/amikacin, an active regimen that can be given once a day, reduces cost substantially as compared to the administration of the same regimen within the hospital. In addition, in those patients who can take oral antibiotics (amoxicillin/clavulanate and ciprofloxacin) the costs can be reduced further : 43 US dollars, including daily surveillance at home by a physician and a nurse.

As indicated in Table 9, the use of G-CSF is not very cost effective for the prevention of febrile neutropenia. In a recent meta-analysis by Messori et al. (12), the average cost associated with the prevention of one episode of neutropenic fever was 14 372 US dollars using the Italian price of the drug converted to dollars and 41 088 dollars using the US price. It is possible, but not proven, that this cost effectiveness might be better in patients with prolonged neutropenia.

On the other hand, as indicated in Table 10, the addtion of GM-CSF or G-CSF to antibiotics for the treatment of febrile neutropenia is associated with a significantly more rapid recovery of adequate neutrophil counts and a significantly reduced duration of hospitalization. In the 2 studies summarized in Table 10 (14, 15) there was a substantial reduction of the cost in the patients receiving the granulopoietic growth factor as compared to a placebo.

The subgroups of patients likely to benefit most from the use of these factors in established febrile neutropenia remain to be defined; in Mitchell's study (14) patients with ALL benefited more than those with solid tumors, supporting Schimpff's recommendation to use therapeutically GM-CSF or G-CSF in those patients with expected prolonged ans severe neutropenia (18).

The prophylactic use of antibiotics for the prevention of febrile neutropenia is a disputed approach because of the risk of emergence of resistance (23). A recent meta analysis by Cruciani et al. (19) showed that prophylaxis was effective in preventing both Gram positive and Gram negative bacteremia in 20 % of the treated patients. As indicated in Table 12, it can be seen that prophylaxis in patients treated with high dose chemotherapy might be modestly cost beneficial but it would not be in patients treated with standard dose chemotherapy.

On the basis of the preceeding considerations, an algorithm for the treatment of febrile neutropenia, that takes into account the cost-benefit, is proposed as indicatived in Table 13, as an incentive to further clinical studies aimed to its validation or rejection.

Table 13
An algorithm for therapy of febrile neutropenia
taking into account cost effectiveness

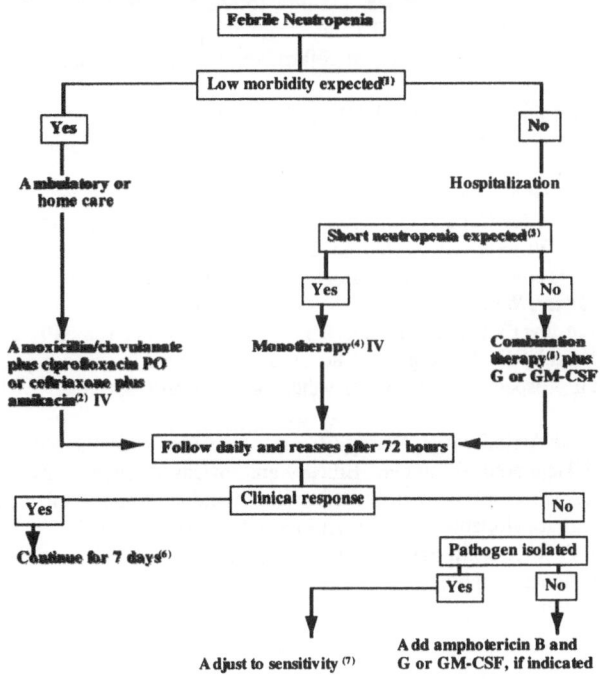

52

(1) Talcott's group IV
(2) Once daily administration possible
(3) cf Blay et al.
(4) Ceftazidime, cefepime, imipenem, meropenem, piperacillin-tazobactam
(5) cf monotherapy plus aminoglycosides
(6) Aminoglycoside to be discontinued after 72 hours if no evidence of Gram negative bacillary bacteremia; G or GM-CSF to be discontinued if neutrophil count > 1000 x cu mm
(7) Glycopeptide for Gram positive bacteremia

References

1. Bodey GP. The treatment of febrile neutropenia from the dark ages to the present. Support Care Cancer 1997, 5 : 351-357.
2. EORTC International Antimicrobial Therapy Cooperative Group. Ceftazidime combined with a short or long course of amikacin for empirical therapy of gram-negative bacteremia in cancer patients with granulocytopenia. N Eng J Med 1987, 317 : 1692-1698.
3. EORTC International Antimicrobial Therapy Cooperative Group. Monotherapy with meropenem versus combination therapy with ceftazidime plus amikacin as empiric therapy for fever in granulocytopenic patients with cancer. Antimicrob Agents Chemother 1995, 40 : 1108-1115.
4. Freifeld AG, Walsh T, Marshall D et al. Monotherapy for fever and neutropenia in cancer patients : a randomized comparison of ceftazidime versus imipenem. J Clin Oncol 1995, 13 : 165-176.
5. Elting LS, Rubenstein EB, Rolston KVI et al. Outcomes of bacteremia in patients with cancer and neutropenia : observations from two decades of epidemiological clinical trials. Clin Infect Dis 1997, 25 : 247-59.
6. Europen Organization for Research and Treatment of Cancer (EORTC) International Antimicrobial Therapy Cooperative Group and the National Cancer Institute of Canada - Clinical Trials Groups. Vancomycin added to empirical combination antibiotic therapy for fever in granulocytopenic cancer patients. J Infect Dis 1991, 163 : 951-958.
7. Rubin M, Hathorn JW, Marshall D et al. Gram-positive infections and the use of vancomycin in 550 episodes of fever and neutropenia. Ann Intern Med 1988, 108 : 30-35.
8. Talcott JA, Siegel RD, Finberg R et al. Risk assessment in cancer patients with fever and neutropenia : a prospective, two-center validation of a prediction rule. J Clin Oncol 1992, 10 : 316-322.
9. The International Antimicrobial Therapy Cooperative Group of the European Organization for Research and Treatment of Cancer. Efficacy and toxicity of single daily doses of amikacin and ceftriaxone versus multiple daily doses of amikacin and ceftazidime for infection in patients with cancer and granulocytopenia. Ann Intern Med 1993, 119 : 584-593.
10. Sundararajan V, Rubenstein EB, Rolston KVI et al. Controversies in new antibiotic therapy for ambulatory patients. Support Care Cancer 1997, 5 : 358-364.

11. Hartmann LC, Tschetter LK, Habermann TM et al. Granulocyte colony stimulating factor in severe chemotherapy induced afebrile neutropenia. New Engl J Med 1997, 336 : 1776-80.

12. Messori A, Trippoli S, Tendi E. G-CSF for the prophylaxis of neutropenic fever in patients with small cell lung cancer receiving myelosuppressive antineoplastic chemotherapy : meta-analysis and pharmacoeconomic evaluation. J Clin Pharmacy & Ther 1996, 21 : 57-63.

13. Geissler K, Koller E, Hubmann E et al. Granulocyte colony-stimulating factor as an adjunct to induction chemotherapy for adult acute lymphoblastic leukemia : a randomized phase III study. Blood 1997, 90 : 590-596.

14. Mitchell PLR, Morland B Stevens MCG et al. Granulocyte colony-stimulating factor in established febrile neutropenia : a randomized study of pediatric patients. J Clin Oncol 1997, 15 : 1163-1170.

15. Maher DW, Lieschke GJ, Green M et al. Filgrastim in patients with chemotherapy-induced febrile neutropenia. Ann Intern Med 1994, 121 : 492-501.

16. Vellenga E, Uyl-de Groot CA, de Wit R et al. Randomized placebo-controlled trial of granulocyte-macrophage colony-stimulating factor in patients with chemotherapy-related febrile neutropenia. J Clin Oncol 1996, 14 : 619-627.

17. Anaissie EJ, Vartivarian S, Bodey GP et al. Randomized comparison between antibiotics alone and antibiotics plus granulocyte-macrophage colony-stimulating factor (Escherichia coli-delivered) in cancer patients with fever and neutropenia. Am J Med 1995, 100 : 17-23.

18. Schimpff SC. Growth factors and empiric therapy with antibiotics : should they be used concurrently ? Ann Intern Med 1994, 121 : 538-540.

19. Cruciani M, Rampazzo R, Malena M et al. Prophylaxis with fluoroquinolones for bacterial infections in neutropenic patients : a meta-analysis. Clin Infect Dis 1996, 23 : 795-805.

20. Blay JY, Chauvin F, Le Cesne A et al. Early lymphopenia after cytotoxic chemotherapy as a risk factor for febrile neutropenia. J Clin Oncol 1996, 14 : 636-643.

21. Rossi C, Klastersky J. Initial empirical antibiotic therapy for neutropenic fever: analysis of the causes of death. Support Care Cancer 1996, 4 : 207-212.

22. Klastersky J. Treatment of neutropenic infection : trends towards monotherapy ? Support Care Cancer 1997, 5 : 365-370.

23. Murphy M, Brown AE, Sepkowitz KA et al. Fluoroquinolone prophylaxis for the prevention of bacterial infections in patients with cancer - is it justified ? Clin Infect Dis 1997, 25 : 346-7.

Alleviation of Dyspnea in Patients with Advanced Cancer : Usefulness of Opioid

Yasuo Shima [1]
Ryusei Saito [2]

1 Palliative Care Unit , National Cancer Center Hospital East, 6-5-1 Kashiwanoha, Kashiwa,Chiba,277-0827 Japan

2 Palliative Care Unit, National Nshigunma Hospital, 2854 Kanai, Shibukawa, Gunma,377-0027 Japan

SUMMARY. We report two studies to evaluate the effectiveness of systemic opioid as symptomatic treatment of dyspnea in patients with advanced cancer. In the first study, the severity of dyspnea was reduced by at least one grade in 15(71%) of the 21 patients and was not reduced in 6(29%).The average dose of morphine was 32.2 mg.In another study, the protocol was prepared collaboratively by the palliative care team of 2 istitutions. Improvement rates were similar in the 2 institutions; 76% and 68%. We suggest that small starting dose of morphine should be given for dyspnea and then gradually increased. Patients should be advised about side-effect and carefully monitored.

KEY WORDS: Dyspnea, Morphine, Treatment ,Effectiveness,Adverse effects

INTRODUCTION

Dyspnea is a patient's subjective symptom, in a strict meaning, and subjective feeling to
require effort in respiration. Dyspnea appearing with progress of cancer in one of the most frequent symptoms from which patients suffer equal to pain.But it is also one of the more poorly understood areas of palliative medical practice. The understanding and management of pain in advanced cancer has been central to the development of palliative care as a science and a humanistic medical care discipline. Oral morphine is widely used as treatment of pain in patients with advanced cancer.
Some health professionals fear that the respiratory depressant effects of morphine will hasten death and induce respiratory failure. However, opioid-induced respiratory suppression did not find in a group of cancer patients who were fully pain controlled on a stable dose of oral morphine.We carried out a pilot study and an open, uncontrolled study to evaluate the effectiveness and the safety of morphine as symptomatic treatment of dyspnea in patients with advanced cancer.

I. Pilot study

Methods ; Patients with dyspnea, either at rest or on exertion , associated with primary and / or secondary malignant intra-thoracic disease under the care of palliative care unit, National Cancer Center Hospital East, between July 1992 and June 1993 entered the trial. Patients were eligible if they had : (1) no reversible causes for breathlessness diagnosed from their history, clinical examination ; (2) no documented renal failure ; (3) no confusion or dementia ; (4) no chemotherapy and / or radiotherapy in the preceding week ; (5) no drainage of pleural effusion in the preceding week ; (6) no course of antibiotics in the preceding week ; (7) no increase in corticosteroids in the preceding week ; (8) no change in other regular medication in the preceding 48h. All patients gave informed consent. Morphine was first administered in a dose of 3mg 4 times daily in a aqueous solution. The dose was then increased by 1 mg.

Dyspnea was assessed using the Dyspnea Evaluation Flow-sheets (DEF) and 4 grades of a Verbal Rating Scare (VRS), "none", "mild", "moderate" and "severe". Dysnea was observed using skin oxygen saturation measured by pulse oxymeter, from the pulse rate, respiration rate and the presence or absence of cyanosis.

Result ; In this study, 21 patients with far-advanced cancer were enrolled. As a result, the severity of dyspnea was reduced by at least one grade in 15(71%) of the 21 patients and was not reduced in 6(29%). The average dose of morphine was 32.2 mg.

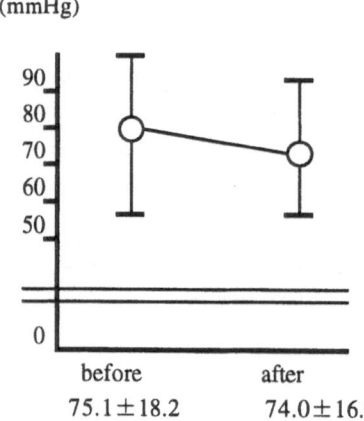

(mmHg)

	before	after
	75.1±18.2	74.0±16.8

Fig.1. Comparison of P$_{O_2}$ before / after Morphine Administration (N=18)

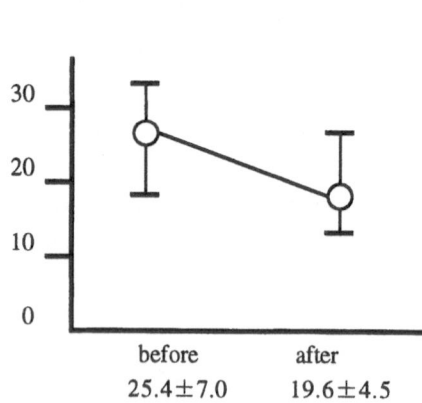

(times)

	before	after
	25.4±7.0	19.6±4.5

Fig.2. Comparison of Respiratory rate before / after Morphine Administration(N=18)

Eighteen of the 21 patients were able to be subjected to time-course measurements of respiration rates and skin oxygen saturation using a pulse oxymeter. Skin oxygen saturation was converted into oxygen partial pressure in arterial blood and plotted on a graph. Average oxygen partial pressures before morphine administration were 75.1 ± 18.2 mmHg and were 74.0 ± 16.8 mmHg after morphine administration, with no change seen(Fig.1). Respiration rates decreased before morphine administration from 25.4 ± 7.0 times/minute to 19.6 ± 7.5 times/minute after administration, showing a change(Fig.2). However, administration of morphine was not discontinued in any patients due to suppression of respiration.

Discussion ; Results of the pilot study showed that morphine could be administered safely to patients with dyspnea could be palliated by morphine. From results of the pilot study and other clinical trials, two action mechanisms of morphine in alleviating dyspnea can be assumed in patients with dyspnea as their chief complaint.

First, the respiration rates of patients decreased clearly after the administration of morphine. Consequently, We think that a reduction in oxygen consumption caused by a decrease in respiration rates from the administration of morphine is attributable to the alleviation of dyspnea. In this respect, Moore et al. stated that morphine does not aggravate pulmonary failure, since a reduction in respiration rate caused by the administration of morphine is compensated by respiration reserving ability[1]. Second, no remarkable change in skin oxygen saturation was observed. This result agreed with results reported by Cohen et al.[2]. We think, therefore, that the alleviation of dyspnea achieved through the administration of morphine is not correlated with results concerning arterial blood gases. Rather, We think that morphine works on the center, such as the cerebral cortex, to exert an effect to lower levels of discomforts.

II. Opened clinical trial

Methods ; A prospective open clinical trial was conducted using a common protocol in the palliative care unit (PCU) of the National Cancer Center Hospital East (NCCH East) and the PCU of the National Nishigunma Hospital (NNH) during a period from April 1994 to May 1996.
The protocol was prepared collaboratively by the palliative care team of the NCCH East and the NNH. Patient eligibility criteria is the same as protocol of the pilot study in the PCU of the NCCH East. Severities of dyspnea were evaluated using 5 grades of verbal rating score (VRS),"None","Mild","Moderate","Severe","Unbearable", referring to the result of the pilot study. Theraputic effects were evaluated as "extremely effective" when dyspnea was alleviated for 2 or more grades or when dyspnea disappeared completely, and "effective" when dyspnea was alleviated for 1 grade.

Table.1.   Administration of Morphine for Dyspnea

1. Oral administration
   · Morphine solution at dose of : 3mg → 5mg → 7mg → 10mg.......
   · frequency of administration : every 4-6hours
2. Continuous subcutaneous infusion
   · Morphine injection at a rate of : 0.5mg / hr → 1.0mg/hr......
   · 24-hour continuous infusion
3. Increasing dosage
   · Targeting a respiratory rate of about 20 times / min. Careful administration should
     be made in the case of ≦10times / min.
   · Range of increasing dosage : 20-50% of the dose

Morphine was administered according to the fixed regimen (Table. 1). The starting dose of morphine was 3mg for oral administration. Continuous subcutaneous infusion was started at 0.5mg/hour. Doses of morphine were increased in units of 20~50% and respiration rates were observed continuously until the dyspnea was alleviated. When morphine was administered a dose that was 20~50% higher the previous dose   was used.

Table.2. Patient Background

	NCCH East PCU (N=48)	NNH PCU (N=56)
Average age (years)	62.2	65.3
Sex(male/female)	21 / 26	33 / 23
Disease	20 / 9 / 19	28 / 12 / 16
(Lung cancer / bresast cancer / other)		

Result ; According to the eligibility criteria, 48 and 56 patients with chief complaints of dyspnea were registered the PCU of the NCCH East and the PCU of the NNH.

Patients with primary lung cancer accounted for the majority, 42% and 50%, in respective hospitals (Table. 2). The causes of dyspnea were classified as follows, pulmonary, where causes reside in the lungs, and non-pulmonary, where the causes reside outsides the lungs. Pulmonary causes were further classified into reduction in the respiratory area due to enlargement of lung tumors, pleural effusion, etc., and airway obstruction. A reduction in the respiratory area occurred frequently among causes of dyspnea in patients registered in the two institutions. A total of enlargement of lung tumors and retention of pleural effusion accounted for 74% in the PCU of the NCCH East and 57% in the PCU of the NNH.

The severity of dyspnea, before administration morphine were mild in 39%,moderate in 34%,sever in 25% and unbearable in 1%.These figures were completely the same in both institutions. Results showed that patients with mild and moderate dyspnea amounted to the majority with the administration of morphine starting.

Table.3.Treatment Effects of Morphine Administration (%)

	NCCH East PCU (N=48)		NNH PCU (N=56)	
Extremely effective	30	(62)	30	(54)
Effective	7	(14)	8	(14)
Not effective	2	(5)	8	(14)
Not evaluable	9	(17)	10	(18)
	48	(100)	56	(100)

Therapeutic effects in patients registered in the 2 institutions were evaluated
according to the criteria. (Table.3) Improvement rates including patients attaining "extremely effective" and "effective" results were similar in the 2 institutions; 76% in the PCU of the NCCH East and 68% in the PCU of the NNH . Therapeutic effect could not be evaluated in 17 % and 18 % of patients due to poor general conditions in the respective institutions.

Medians of the first dosages of morphine were 30 mg and 24 mg and the medians of the maximum dosages were 57 mg and 48 mg in the respective institutions. It took 3.5 days on average to alleviate dyspnea in both institutions. Dyspnea was alleviated within a short period of time, 3~4 days,by administering morphine and indicates that morphine exerted its therapeutic effect swiftly.

Table.4. Adverse Effects with Morphine Administration(%)

	NCCH East PCU (N=48)		NNH PCU (N=56)	
Nausea and vomitting	8	(17)	8	(14)
Drowsiness	5	(10)	5	(9)
Constipation	20	(42)	10	(18)
Respiratory suppression	0	(0)	0	(0)

Nausea, vomiting and constipation occurred frequently as adverse effects of morphine in both institutions (Table. 4). Drowsiness was observed in 10% and 9% of the patients in the respective institutions. In patients complaining of drowsiness a reduction in respiration rate was also observed and controlling measures, such as reducing dosage, were conducted. Drowsiness therefore was important among the adverse effects, since it was a prodrome of respiration suppression. If drowsiness occurs, patients should be monitored carefully and the dose adjusted. A remarkable reduction in respiration rate was not observed.

Discussion ; Our results suggest that morphine will give symptomatic relief in some dyspneic patients with advanced cancer. Unfortunately, due to open and uncontrolled study, the level of evidence was not enough. This is a common problem for clinical studies in palliative medicine and highlights the needs for randomized controlled trials[3].

In the case of cancer-related dyspnea, all the published studies have agreed on the beneficial effect of systemic opioids for dyspnea. However, the optimal type, dose, and modality of administration of opioid has not yet been determined. In addition, adverse effects of systemic opioids for dyspnea is also unclear. Bruera et al. conducted two trials using intermittent subcutaneous morphine for the relief of dyspnea[4.5]. In the first study, intermittent doses of up to 2.5 times the regular opioid dose resulted in no significant change in the end-tidal CO_2 level in these patients. On the other hand, results of our pilot study showed that there were not significantly change between average oxygen partial pressures before morphine administration and after morphine administration. These results may have been because most of patients already had been chronically exposed to opioids and therefore had developed tolerance to their respiratory depressant effect.

The high incidence of adverse effect, particularly drowsiness and sedation, was of concern and indicates a need to monitor these patients carefully. Previous studies have demonstrated transient cognitive impairment, including sedation, following opioid dose increase in patients with cancer pain[6]. It was reassuring to find that there was no clinically significant deterioration in respiratory function despite the very poor baseline levels of patients with advanced cancer. We suggest that small starting dose of morphine should be given for dyspnea and then gradually increased. Patients ought to be advised about potential side-effect and adequate supervision arranged particularly for medical stuff. Doses should be titrated in individual patients against response and side-effects and other symptomatic treatments as an alternative to morphine or in combination with it.

A common clinical impression in palliative care of cancer patient is that many patients are dyspneic intermittently, usually in relation to excertion, obstruction of air ways with mucus, or psychological factors. Therefore the use of intermittent opioids would seen more logical for breathlessness than chronic regular doing in these patients. We think that it is necessary to positively consider administrating intermittent 'as required' opioids before dyspnea becomes severe. The nebulized route of delivering opioids may prove to be a most fruitful line of research and development, as it offers the following; speed of effect and reduced systemic side-effect. Most immportantly, the patient has the opportunity to regulate his own medication on a 'as require' basis, so minimizing drug intake while bestowing autonomy[7]. However, there remains a lot of problems to be solved. To give an example, the problem is to determine adequate doses and adequate administration intervals. The design of study is especially in the study of treatment using the nebulized route of delivering opioids. We think it is necessary to conduct double blind randomized controlled trials of nebulized opioids.

REFERENCES

1. Moore DP, Weston AR, Hughes JMB, et al. (1992) Effects of increased inspired oxygen concentrations on exercise performance in chronic heart failure. Lancet 339:850-853

2. Cohen MH, Johnston Anderson A, Krasnow SH, et al. (1991) Continuous intravenous infusion of morphine for severe dyspnea. South Med J 84: 229-234

3. Cook DJ, Guyatt GH, Laupacis A, et al. (1992) Rules of evidence and clinical recommendations on the use of antithrombotic agents. Chest 102: 205S-311S

4. Bruera E, MacEachern T, Ripamonti C, et al. (1993) Subcutaneous morphine for dyspnea in cancer patients. Ann Intern Med 119: 906-907

5. Bruera E, Macmillan K, Pither J, et al. (1990) The effects of morphine on dyspnea of terminal cancer patients. J Pain Sympt Manag 5:341-344

6. Bruera E, Macmillan K, Hanson J, et al. (1989) The cognitive effects of the administration of narcotic analgesics in patients with cancer pain. Pain 39:13-16

7. Ahmedzai S. (1998) Palliation of respiratory symptoms. In: Doyle D, Hanks GWC, MacDonald RN(eds)Oxford textbook of palliative medicine,2nd ed. Oxford University Press ,Oxford,pp583-616

Symptom Control in Palliative Medicine: Standard Management and Clinical Trials II

Fumikazu Takeda, MD, Chairman of the session

After introductory remarks by the chairman, Dr. Geert H Blijham, The Netherlands, Prof. Feld discussed the frequency, causes and management of chronic nausea in patients with advanced cancer. He stated that estimates of frequency of nausea in terminal cancer patients are as high as 50 to 60% with more females exhibiting this symptom, vomiting is manifested by about 30% of patients and certain cancer may be predisposed to this problem. Citing from the study results which were reported by Bruera and his colleagues and others, Prof. Feld addressed cause and treatment of chronic nausea in patients with advanced cancer. It may be specifically due to dysfunction of the autonomic nervous system manifested by delayed gastric emptying. It is often associated with anorexia and weight loss. In order to assume that chronic nausea in advanced cancer is present, all possible causes of nausea such as metabolic causes, side-effects of cancer therapies and drugs, brain metastasis, GI tract obstruction, etc. must be ruled out. General measures such as small meal portions, low fat meals and exclusion of dairy related foods and spicy foods may help. Controlled release metoclopramide is safe and effective in managing chronic nausea in patients with advanced cancer, If nausea is not fully controlled, he recommends to alternatively use dexamethasone, then, haloperidol, dimenhydranate and cisapride. Recently, megestrol acetate were reported to be effective. Discussion included that further studies are needed to better define the relative contribution of each of the potential causes and factors, since very little is known about this problem, and that prospective comparative clinical trials of different antiemetics should be conducted.

Prof. Klastersky discussed management strategies of infection in neutropenic patients. Over the past two decades, Gram-positive infections have increased and Gram-negative infections have progressively become a less frequent causes of sepsis in neutropenic patients, currently accounting for only 30% of infections. He discussed the latest antimicrobial management against Gram-negative as well as Gram-positive bacterial infections, and the use of antifungal agents when patient remains neutropenic and febrile and initial microbiological workup has been negative, especially in patients with severe neutropenia and/or a newly apparent clinical site of infection. He also mentioned of antimicrobial treatment in patients who are immunosuppressed, such as those with graft-versus-host disease after allogeneic bone marrow transplantation. Indication of the use of colony stimulating factor was also discussed. It can be used as an adjunct to antibacterial and antifungal agents when neutropenia is severe and the control of infection is not optimal. Alternative role of preemptive and prophylactic therapies need to be clearly defined. It was also addressed to provide support for infectious complications more often at home and within an ambulatory settings.

Usefulness and effectiveness of opioid drugs in the relief of dyspnea was discussed by Dr. Shima. Dyspnea, a subjective symptom and a subjective sensation requiring respiratory effort, frequently develops in patients with terminal cancer. It was found in 21% of the patients at their admission to the Palliative Care Unit of the National Cancer Center Hospital East in Kashiwa, Japan. Such dyspnea is usually so severe that it may induce the patient's and caregivers' anxieties and fears that the patient's death is impending. Dr. Shima revealed that morphine administration (by mouth in most cases) was effective in three-fourths of 56 patients with dyspnea. The initial dose of morphine was 74.9mg per day in average and the dose at the maximum was 149.3mg in average. The number of days required for alleviation of the dyspnea was 3.5 days in average. In his another study, Dr. Shima revealed that the rate of breathing decreased significantly with the morphine administration, but the PaO$_2$ before the treatment was 75.1Å}18.2, whereas it was 74.0Å}16.8 after the morphine administration. This clearly demonstrates safety and effectiveness of rational morphine use in the relief of dyspnea in terminally-ill cancer patients. He suggests that reduced oxygen consumption induced by decreased breathing rate due to morphine administration contributes to relief of dyspnea. It was also discussed that dyspnea should be always relieved of in order to ease the suffering of the patient himself/herself as well as to ease the anxieties and fears of his/her care-givers.

Session III

Depression:
A Major Psychological and
Emotional Problem

Chairpersons:
Eduardo Bruera and Shigeto Yamawaki

DEPRESSION IN PATIENTS WITH ADVANCED CANCER

Hitoshi Okamura[1], Tatsuo Akechi[2], Akira Kugaya[2], Ichiro Mikami[2,3], Toru Okuyama[2], Tomohito Nakano[2], Ariyuki Kagaya[3], Shigeto Yamawaki[3] and Yosuke Uchitomi[2]

[1]Department of Psychiatry, National Cancer Center Hospital, 5-1-1 Tsukiji, Chuo-ku, Tokyo, 104 Japan. [2]Psycho-Oncology Division, National Cancer Center Research Institute East, Kashiwa, 277 Japan. [3]Department of Psychiatry and Neurosciences, Hiroshima University School of Medicine, Hiroshima, 734 Japan

SUMMARY. Prevalence and risk factors for depression, desire for death, and diagnosing depression were examined in patients with advanced cancer. 1) Of 141 subjects, 44 patients diagnosed with recurrent breast cancer and 97 with advanced non-small-cell lung cancer, 43.2% of those with recurrent breast cancer and 14.4% of those with advanced non-small-cell lung cancer met the DSM-III-R criteria for adjustment disorder or major depression. Logistic regression analysis showed that a disease-free interval less than 24 months in recurrent breast cancer and low fighting spirit, family history of cancer death, past history of depression and dissatisfaction with confidants in non-small-cell lung cancer significantly predicted a diagnosis of adjustment disorder or major depression. These results indicate that psychosocial interventions are necessary for patients with advanced cancer who have risk factors for depression. 2) All of 5 patients with terminal cancer who expressed a desire for death were diagnosed with major depression according to DSM-III-R. After treatment with tricyclic antidepressants, they all showed remarkable improvement of depressed mood and their desire for death had almost disappeared. These experiences suggest that appropriate treatment of depression may alter the desire for death in terminally ill cancer patients. However, depression is frequently underdiagnosed and undertreated because the diagnostic criteria of major depression include physical symptoms normally observed during the course of cancer and/or cancer treatment. We propose using a biological marker (serotonin2A receptor-mediated Ca^{2+} response in human platelets) as one of the adjuncts in diagnosing depression in cancer patients.

KEY WORDS: depression, DSM-III-R, advanced cancer, desire for death, serotonin2A receptor-mediated Ca^{2+} response

INTRODUCTION

Depression including adjustment disorder and major depression is frequently observed in cancer patients. It has been reported that prevalence rates of depression in patients with advanced cancer range from 20% [1] to more than 40% [2]. This variation in the prevalence reflects differences in assessment tools, definition of depression, time since diagnosis, and disease site or stage; most of the reports have assessed depression using rating scales, not structured clinical interviews. Therefore, we initially investigated the prevalence of depression in patients with recurrent breast cancer and advanced non-small-cell lung cancer using structured clinical interviews to evaluate diagnostic criteria at a fixed interval after diagnosis.

With regard to risk factors for depression in cancer patients, Breitbart [3] reported the following four factors: cancer-related factors (for example, the presence of pain), cancer treatment-related factors, psychiatric history, and social factors (for example, absence of social support). However, there are no reports in patients with advanced cancer. Second, we examined predictive factors for depression in patients with recurrent breast cancer and advanced non-small-cell lung cancer.

Recently, depression in terminally ill cancer patients has been discussed in association with euthanasia or physician-assisted suicide. While it has been reported that a desire for death is closely associated with depression [4,5], there are few useful reports concerning the 'treatability' of depression under such conditions. Third, we report previously encountered patients with terminal cancer who expressed a desire for death and responded to general antidepressant treatment.

As previously mentioned, diagnosing depression accurately is very important; however, it is difficult to detect depression in cancer patients, because the diagnostic criteria for major depression includes neurovegetative symptoms that can be attributed to cancer and/or cancer treatment (e.g., appetite loss, insomnia, fatigue, and diminished ability to concentrate). Objective markers would be helpful in diagnosing depression in these patients. Therefore, we propose using a biological marker as an adjunct in diagnosing depression in cancer patients.

PREVALENCE AND RISK FACTORS FOR DEPRESSION IN PATIENTS WITH ADVANCED CANCER

Patients and methods

Forty-four patients with recurrent breast cancer who met the eligibility criteria shown in Table 1, and 97 with advanced non-small-cell lung cancer who met the eligibility criteria shown in Table 2 participated in the study. This study was carried out three months after the diagnosis in those with recurrent breast cancer, and between admission and initial treatments in those with advanced non-small-cell lung cancer.

Table 1. Eligibility criteria in recurrent breast cancer

I-1. Eligibility criteria
   1) histologically or cytologically documented breast cancer and histologically, cytologically or clinically proven recurrence of breast cancer
   2) age greater than 15 years
   3) an Eastern Cooperative Oncology Group (ECOG) performance status is 0 to 3
   4) written informed consent is obtained

I-2. Exclusion criteria
   1) patients with severe physical conditions
   2) patients with an active concomitant malignancy
   3) patients with clouding of consciousness

Table 2. Eligibility criteria in advanced non-small-cell lung cancer

---

I-1. Eligibility criteria
   1) histologically or cytologically documented non-small-cell lung cancer
   2) clinical stage: III or IV
   3) age greater than 18 years
   4) written informed consent is obtained

I-2. Exclusion criteria
   1) patients with severe physical conditions
   2) patients with brain metastasis
   3) patients with cognitive impairment

Adjustment disorder and major depression in these subjects were assessed according to the Structured Clinical Interview for DSM-III-R [6] (SCID). In addition, the participants were asked to complete the Profile of Mood States (POMS) [7] which assesses 6 emotional states and total mood disturbance, and the Mental Adjustment to Cancer (MAC) scale [8] which assesses the specific mental adjustment (coping) of cancer patients.

Risk factors including demographic, medical, and psychosocial variables were analyzed using the logistic regression model. Data analyses were carried out with SAS statistical software (SAS Institute Inc., 1997).

Results

Demographic, medical and psychosocial data for 44 patients with recurrent breast cancer and 97 with advanced non-small-cell lung cancer are summarized in Table 3.

Table 3. Demographic, medical and psychosocial characteristics

	Recurrent breast cancer N (%)	Non-small-cell lung cancer N (%)
Total	44 (100)	97 (100)
Gender		
M	0	72 (74.2)
F	44 (100)	25 (25.8)
Age		
Median	50.8	64.0
Mean ($\pm$ SD)	49.5$\pm$ 9.7	62.9$\pm$ 8.4
Education		
$\leq$ 12 years	25 (56.8)	76 (78.4)
> 12 years	19 (43.2)	21 (21.6)

Table 3. Demographic, medical and psychosocial characteristics (Continued)

	Recurrent breast cancer N (%)	Non-small-cell lung cancer N (%)
Marital status		
Married	36 (81.8)	83 (85.6)
Unmarried	8 (18.2)	14 (14.4)
Employment status		
Employed	19 (43.2)	31 (32.0)
Unemployed	25 (56.8)	66 (68.0)
Performance status		
0 , 1, 2	43 (97.7)	94 (96.9)
3, 4	1 (2.3)	3 (3.1)
Pain		
Presence	18 (40.9)	45 (46.4)
Absence	26 (59.1)	52 (53.6)
No. of confidants		
0, 1, 2	13 (29.5)	49 (50.5)
≥ 3	31 (70.5)	48 (49.5)
Satisfaction with confidants		
dissatisfaction	12 (27.3)	16 (16.5)
satisfaction	32 (72.7)	81 (83.5)
Coping style		
Fighting spirit		
Median	46.5	49.0
Mean (± SD)	47.5± 8.3	48.4± 7.5
Helplessness/hopelessness		
Median	10.0	11.0
Mean (± SD)	10.8± 3.9	11.1± 3.7
Disease free interval		
< 24 months	14 (31.8)	-
≥ 24 months	30 (68.2)	-

Of these subjects, 43.2% in recurrent breast cancer and 14.4% in advanced non-small-cell lung cancer met the DSM-III-R criteria for adjustment disorder or major depression. Adjustment disorder was seen in 16 (36.4%) and 13 (13.4%), and major depression in 3 (6.8%) and 1 (1.0 %), respectively.

We used multivariate logistic regression to examine independent risk factors of depression, on the basis of possible factors according to univariate analysis. Logistic regression analysis showed that a disease-free interval less than 24 months in recurrent breast cancer and low fighting spirit, family history of cancer death, past history of depression and dissatisfaction with confidants in advanced non-small-cell lung cancer significantly predicted a diagnosis of adjustment disorder or major depression (Table 4).

Table 4. Risk factors for depression -Logistic regression analysis-

	Demographic factors	Medical factors	Psychosocial factors
Recurrent breast cancer		short disease-free interval* (< 24 months)	
Non-small-cell lung cancer	family history of cancer death**		low fighting spirit* past history of depression* dissatisfaction with confidants*

**p<0.01, *p<0.05

DESIRE FOR DEATH IN PATIENTS WITH ADVANCED CANCER

Between October 1996 and May 1997, we encountered 5 patients with terminal cancer who expressed a desire for death and were referred to the Department of Psychiatry, National Cancer Center. All of the patients were diagnosed with major depression according to DSM-III-R. Approximately one week after treatment with tricyclic antidepressants, they all showed remarkable improvement of depressed mood and their desire for death had almost disappeared. We present one of these 5 patients, and summarize the data from all 5 patients in Table 5.

Case

A 58-year-old man was admitted to the palliative care unit to manage his general fatigue, nausea, and digestive disturbances. He had received a diagnosis of pancreatic cancer 6 months earlier, and carcinomatous peritonitis had recently developed. Despite various attempts of symptomatic management, these symptoms persisted. Three weeks after admission, psychiatric referral was made by his attending physician, because the patient expressed a strong desire for death and requested sedation. On the initial interview, the patient complained of irritation and discussed the idea of suicide. His mood was depressed and psychomotor retardation was recognized. The score on the Hamilton Rating Scale for Depression was 54. We diagnosed the patient major depression according to the DSM-III-R and began to administer a tricyclic antidepressant, clomipramine at a dose of 75 mg daily. One week after the treatment, his depressed mood was remarkably improved, and the patient did not express any further desire for death or sedation. The score of Hamilton Rating Scale for Depression reduced to 16. He appeared to have a better quality of life untill the end.

With regard to treatment of major depression in cancer patients, we developed an algorithm for the treatment (Figure 1) and its feasibility is now under investigation [9].

DIAGNOSING DEPRESSION IN CANCER PATIENTS BY A BIOLOGICAL MARKER

Blood samples were drawn from a control (57 years old, male, lung cancer, stage I, performance status=0) and a depressed patient (59 years old, male, lung cancer, stage IIa, performance status=0), from whom informed consent was obtained. The serotonin (5-HT)-stimulated increase

Table 5. Summary of 5 cancer patients who complained of an expressed desire for death

Sex	Age	Primary cancer site	Treatment	Hamilton Rating Scale for Depression*	
				Before	1 week after treatment
F	68	lung	amitriptyline (PO)	24	10
M	72	stomach	amitriptyline (IV)	34	17
M	58	pancreas	clomipramine (IV)	54	16
F	58	sigmoid colon	clomipramine (IV)	35	16
M	53	lung	clomipramine (IV)	41	12

F: female, M: male, PO: per os, IV: intravenous. * Hamilton Rating Scale for Depression (21 items: 0-64 scores) is a rating scale for the severity of depression.

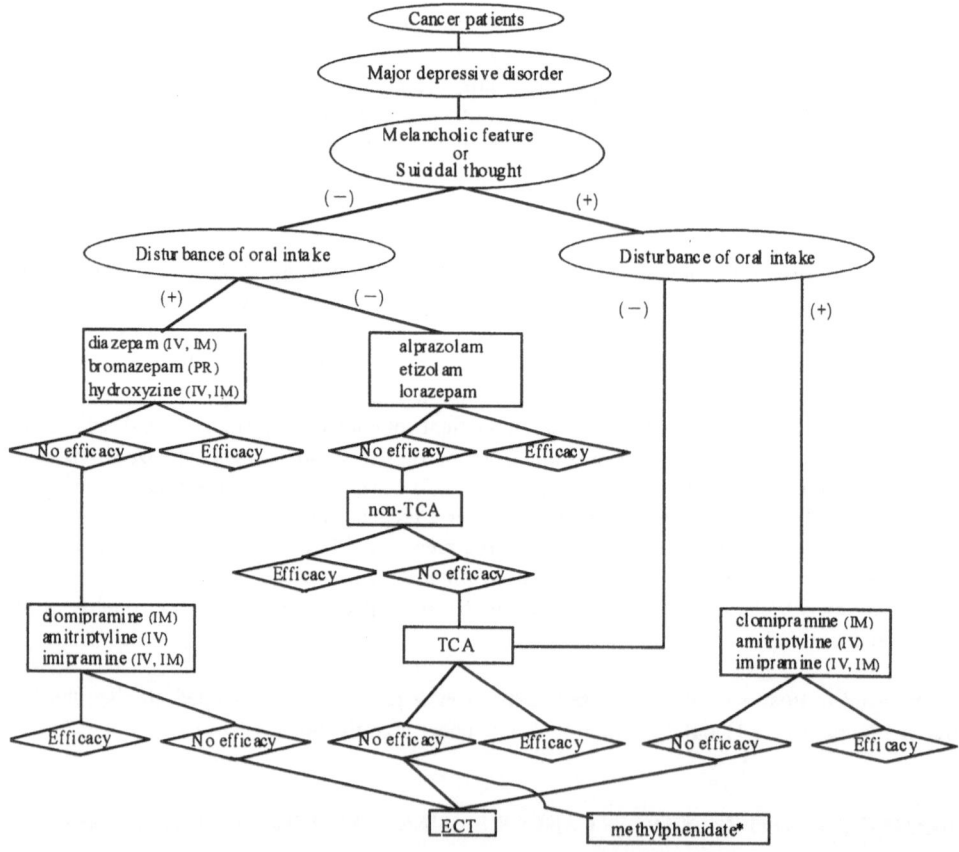

Figure 1. Algorithm for the treatment of major depression in cancer patients. * Recommended for old patients and patients with drowsiness due to narcotics and fatigue due to cachexia.
IV; intravenous, IM; intramuscular, PR; per rectum, TCA; tricyclic antidepressant

in Ca^{2+} in platelets was measured using a fluorescence photometer. Figure 2 shows that the receptor-mediated increase in Ca^{2+} in platelets was significantly enhanced in the depressed patient compared with that in the control.

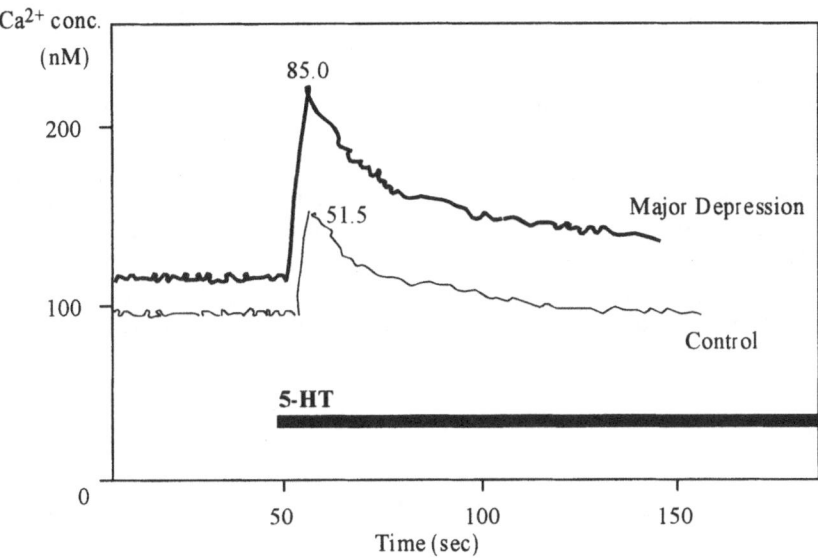

Figure 2. Serotonin-induced platelet Ca^{2+} responses in cancer patients with depression. Transient Ca^{2+} increases after stimulation with serotonin (5-HT) is presented. This figure indicates that the response in the depressed patient is greater than that in the age, gender, and cancer site-matched control (85.0 vs. 51.5 nM).

DISCUSSION

It has been estimated that 25% of cancer patients have clinically significant depressive symptoms or major depression [10,11], and that patients with more advanced cancer have a higher prevalence of depression [12,13]. However, most of the previous studies assessed the prevalence of depression only by rating scales such as Beck Depression Inventory [14] or Hospital Anxiety and Depression Scale [15]. For accurate assessment, it is essential to use structured interviews and standardized diagnostic criteria. The present findings, which were obtained according to the semi-structured interview for DSM-III-R, demonstrated that the prevalence of depression is high in patients with recurrent breast cancer.

Logistic regression analysis showed that a disease-free interval less than 24 months in recurrent breast cancer and low fighting spirit, family history of cancer death, past history of depression and dissatisfaction with confidants in advanced non-small-cell lung cancer significantly predicted a diagnosis of adjustment disorder or major depression. These results indicate that psychosocial interventions are necessary for preventing depression in patients with advanced cancer who demonstrate risk factors for depression.

Our finding that all patients with terminal cancer who expressed a desire for death were diagnosed with major depression is very important when considering the issue of euthanasia or physician-assisted suicide. Many studies also emphasize that depression is common among patients considering euthanasia or physician-assisted suicide [5,16,17] and must be diagnosed as soon as possible [18]. This is because there is a likelihood that depression influences the ability to appreciate life's benefits while magnifying life's burdens [19]. From several surveys, it is thought that if physician-assisted suicide is legalized, physicians will need to gain experience in diagnosing and treating depression as well as in understanding patients' motivations for requesting physician-assisted suicide, maximizing palliative interventions, and evaluating external pressures on the patients [20].

Although research on the efficacy of treatment for depression in terminally ill patients has been limited because of the patients' severe medical condition, all of our cases showed remarkable improvement of depressed mood and their desire for death had almost disappeared one week after treatment with tricyclic antidepressants, as previously reported [21,22]. These results suggest that appropriate treatment for depression can be effective even at the terminal stage, and that the desire for death may be altered in some terminally ill patients after treatment for depression, therefore, such treatments should be considered before justifying euthanasia or physician-assisted suicide.

Table 6. Symptoms of depression according to DSM-III-R diagnostic criteria for major depressive episode

---

(1) depressed mood
(2) diminished interest or pleasure in all, or almost all, and activities
(3) significant weight loss or weight gain when not dieting, or decrease or increase in appetite
(4) insomnia or hypersomnia
(5) psychomotor agitation or retardation
(6) fatigue or loss of energy
(7) feelings of worthlessness or excessive or inappropriate guilt
(8) diminished ability to think or concentrate, or indecisiveness
(9) recurrent thoughts of death, recurrent suicidal ideation without a specific plan, or a suicide attempt or a specific plan for committing suicide

---

However, depression is frequently underdiagnosed and undertreated [23,24] because the diagnostic criteria for major depression (Table 6) includes physical symptoms such as appetite loss, insomnia, fatigue, and diminished ability to concentrate observed during the normal course of cancer and/or cancer treatment. Therefore, many researchers have sought biological markers that could be used as adjuncts in diagnosing depression [25,26]. Abnormality in the 5-HT2 receptor-mediated signaling system is one such marker that has been studied. We have also directed our attention to 5-HT2A receptor-mediated intracellular Ca^{2+} signaling system in depression [27]. Since platelets have 5-HT2 receptors and are thought to be useful peripheral models of signaling systems in the central nervous system, we measured the 5-HT-stimulated increase in Ca^{2+} in platelets. Our results showed that receptor-mediated increase in Ca^{2+} in platelets was significantly enhanced in the depressed patients compared with that in the control. However, we have just started investigations into a useful biological marker, and further investigation is needed.

REFERENCES

1. Hopwood P, Howell A, Maguire P (1991) Screening for psychiatric morbidity in patients with advanced breast cancer : validation of two self-report questionnaires. Br J Cancer 64: 349-352
2. Burkberg J, Penman D, Holland JC (1984) Depression in hospitalized cancer patients. Psychosom Med 46: 199-212
3. Breitbart W (1995) Identifying patients at risk for, and treatment of major psychiatric complications of cancer. Support Care Cancer 3: 45-604.
4. Brown JH, Henteleff P, Barakat S, Rowe CJ (1986) Is it normal for terminally ill patients to desire death?. Am J Psychiatry 143: 208-211
5. Chochinov HM, Wilson KG, Enns M, Mowchun N, Lander S, Levitt M, Clinch JJ (1995) Desire for death in the terminally ill. Am J Psychiatry 152: 1185-1191
6. American Psychiatric Association (1987) Diagnostic and Statistical Manual of Mental Disorders, Third Edition-Revised. American Psychiatric Association, Washington, DC.
7. McNair DM, Lorr M, DroppLemn LF (1971) Manual for the Profile of Mood States (POMS). Educational and Industrial Testing Service, San Diego
8. Watson M, Greer S, Young J, Inayat Q, Burgess C, Robertson B (1988) Development of a questionnaire measure of adjustment to cancer: the MAC scale. Psychol Med 18: 203-209
9. Uchitomi Y, Kugaya A, Akechi T, Nakano T, Okamura H (in press) Algorithms for the treatment of affective disorders: Depression in cancer patients. Jpn J Psychiat Treat
10. Plumb B, Holland JC (1977) Comparative studies of psychological function in patients with advanced cancer I: Self-reported depressive symptoms. Psychosom Med 39: 264-276
11. Evans DL, McCartney CF, Nemeroff CB, Raft D, Quade D, Golden RN, Haggerty JJ Jr, Holmes V, Simon JS, Droba M (1986) Depression in women treated for gynecological cancer: clinical and neuroendocrine assessment. Am J Psychiatry 143: 447-452
12. Cassileth BR, Lusk EJ, Strouse TB, Miller DS, Brown LL, Cross PA, Tenaglia AN (1984) Psychosocial status in chronic illness. A comparative analysis of six diagnostic groups. N Engl J Med 311: 506-511
13. Rodin G, Voshart K (1986) Depression in the medically ill; an overview. Am J Psychiatry 143: 696-705
14. Beck AT, Ward CH, Mendelson M, Mock J, Erbaugh J (1961) An inventory for measuring depression. Arch Gen Psychiatry 4: 561-571
15. Zigmond AS, Snaith RP (1983) The hospital anxiety and depression scale. Acta Psychiatr Scand 67: 361-370
16. Emanuel EJ, Fairclough DL, Daniels ER, Clarridge BR (1996) Euthanasia and physician-assisted suicide: attitudes and experiences of oncology patients, oncologists, and the public. Lancet 347: 1805-1810
17. Breitbart W, Rosenfeld BD, Passik SD (1996) Interest in physician-assisted suicide among ambulatory HIV-infected patients. Am J Psychiatry 153: 238-242
18. Van Der Maas PJ, Van Delden JJ, Pijnenborg L, Looman CW (1991) Euthanasia and other medical decisions concerning the end of life. Lancet 338: 669-674
19. Sullivan MD, Youngner SJ (1994) Depression, competence, and the right to refuse lifesaving medical treatment. Am J Psychiatry 151: 971-978

20. Drickamer MA, Lee MA, Ganzini L (1997) Practical Issues in physician-assisted suicide. Ann Intern Med 126: 146-151.
21. Massie MJ, Holland JC (1990) Depression and cancer patients. J Clin Psychiatry 51: 12-17

22. Woods SW, Tesar GE, Murray GB, Cassem NH (1986) Psychostimulant treatment of depressive disorders secondary to medical illness. J Clin Psychiatry 47: 12-15
23. Derogatis LR, Abeloff MD, McBeth CD (1976) Cancer patients and their physicians in the perception of psychological symptoms. Psychosomatics 17: 197-201
24. Levine PM, Silverfarb PM, Lipowski ZJ (1978) Mental disorders in cancer patients: a study of 100 psychiatric referrals. Cancer. 42: 1385-1391
25. Carroll BJ, Curtis GC, Mendels J (1976) Neuroendocrine regulation in depression : II. Discrimination of depressed from nondepressed patients. Arch Gen Psychiatry 33: 1051-1058
26. Kusumi I, Koyama T, Yamashita I (1994) Serotonin-induced platelet intracellular calcium mobilization in depressed patients. Psychopharmacology 113: 322-327
27. Yamawaki S, Kagaya A, Okamoto Y, Shimizu M, Nishida A, Uchitomi Y (1996) Enhanced calcium response to serotonin in platelets from patients with affective disorders. J Psychiatry Neurosci 21: 321-324

DEPRESSION IN HIV-INFECTED ADULTS: NEWER CONCEPTS

Harry Hollander, M.D.

Professor of Clinical Medicine, Director of Categorical Residency Program, Department of Medicine, University of California, San Francisco, CA 94143, USA

SUMMARY.   HIV infection is commonly accompanied by clinical or subclinical neurological involvement. Thus, it is not surprising that psychological and psychiatric complications of disease are commonly seen.   While suicidality is perhaps less commonly seen than initially thought, depressive symptomatology is common in adults with HIV infection and reflects a complex interplay between biological, psychological, and social factors.   Depression accounts for a significant proportion of somatic symptoms in individuals with early HIV infection, but is most prevalent in people with progressive disease and those who are most disenfranchised. Fortunately, a variety of antidepressants has been demonstrated to ameliorate depressive symptoms in this population, although HIV-infected persons are at higher risk of adverse effects from psychoactive medications. During the past several years, advances in antiretroviral therapy have markedly improved the long term prognosis of HIV disease. These developments have altered the perception of this illness as an invariably terminal disease, but have created new concerns and questions for infected individuals that may cause more short term psychological distress.

KEY WORDS: HIV, depression, substance abuse, pharmacotherapy, improving prognosis

INTRODUCTION

Over the course of the HIV epidemic, a number of assertions regarding the relationship between HIV infection and depression have gained general acceptance, including the following:
1. Depression and suicidality are more prevalent in HIV-infected persons than in the general population or in individuals with other chronic diseases such as cancer.
2. The predominant risk factor for this and other psychiatric complications is a prior history of an axis I diagnosis.
3. The incidence of depression increases as HIV disease progresses in severity.
4. Pharmacologic therapy of depression in this setting is less successful than in other depressed patients.

Many of these conclusions have been based upon data that are significantly flawed. For example, impressions regarding suicide rates were drawn from largely anecdotal reports rather than population-based sampling. Early studies of depression were limited to cohorts from Western nations, often focused on a limited representation of risk and socioeconomic groups, and did not control for an elevated risk of depressive symptoms and depression in uninfected members of the risk groups. Furthermore, methodology of measuring depression has varied markedly between studies, making study to study comparison very difficult.

The study of depression in HIV-infected people is also complicated by the frequent occurrence of primary and secondary central nervous system organic lesions in these individuals. HIV is thought to subclinically infect the nervous system early in the course of disease in a majority of individuals. Over time, the incidence of cognitive impairment increases, and it is currently estimated that approximately 20% of persons with advanced HIV infection (as defined by a CD4 lymphocyte count of less than 200 cells/mm^3) have neurocognitive deficits compatible with the HIV-associated cognitive/motor syndrome (formerly known as the AIDS dementia complex). Early clinical findings of this syndrome may mimic or coexist with depression. Later, patients most commonly exhibit a pattern of subcortical neuropsychiatric deficits, with prominent slowing of processing and associative function, which again may be quite difficult to differetiate from the findings of depression.

In light of all of these issues, the literature in this area must be examined critically. The remainder of this chapter reviews recent data which refine our understanding of this complex psychobiological phenomenon and raises questions about future issues in the context of the changing natural history of HIV infection due to therapeutic advances.

Epidemiology and Risk Factors for Depression

Reports of impressive prevalence of depressive symptoms in selected cohorts of HIV-infected indivduals continue to appear. In a group of 475 seropositive San Francisco men without AIDS, Katz noted that 37% could be classified as depressed based upon a score of 16 or greater on the Center for Epidemiologic Studies Depression scale (CES-D) (1). Utilizing a cut-off of 14 or above on the Beck Depression Inventory (BDI), Judd found a very comparable prevalence of 44% in an outpatient clinic setting in Melbourne (2). Of greater interest are studies which carry out measurements in both infected and uninfected members of the risk groups being studied. In a group of 98 asymptomatic infectected and 71 uninfected homosexual men, Perkins found the lifetime and current prevalence of major depressive disorder to be comparable regardless of serostatus (3). Furthermore, in this cohort, the overall current prevalence of depression of 6% did not greatly exceed estimates in the United States population as a whole. Although different depression scales were used, Rabkin and colleagues reached remarkably similar conclusions in a study of homosexual men (4). Two recent studies have examined the issue of depression in injection drug users. Lipsitz studied over 220 male and female drug users of whom 55% were HIV-infected (5). He found an overall prevalence of depression of 26% in this cohort. Whereas HIV-positive men had a higher rate of depression than HIV-negative men (33% versus 16%), this difference was not observed in the women studied. The WHO Neuropsychiatric AIDS study found a significantly increased score on the Montgomery-Asberg Depression Rating Scale in symptomatic seropositive drug users in Bangkok compared to seronegative controls. This finding was consistent with their results in other risk groups studied in disparate parts of the world (6). Despite the difficulty in directly comparing studies which use different methodologies and endpoints, the recently generated data highlight that underlying behavioral traits, orientation, and socioeconomic status may play an important if not predominant role in determining which HIV-infected persons are at greatest risk for depression. The observation of gender differences within the population of injection drug users also introduces another variable about which little has been written in the past.

In terms of the relationship between the stage of HIV disease and the risk of depression, most cross-sectional studies have suggested an escalating degree of depression during the progression of HIV-related immunosuppression. Two studies convincingly argue that a significant amount of the somatic complaints of fatigue and insomnia in patients with earlier disease and preserved immune function is attributable to depressive symptoms (7,8). In cohorts followed longitudinally, there are conflicting data about whether depressive symptoms increase over time. Rabkin prospectively studied 112 HIV-positive homosexual men over a four year period (9). Compared to HIV-negative controls, these men had a minor increase in somatic depressive symptoms and anxiety throughout the study period. However, despite high rates of HIV disease progression, mean psychopathology symptom scores remained normal and there was no increase in syndromic depression over time. The results from the Multicenter AIDS Cohort Study (MACS) are contradictory (10). In this study, over 900 men who were seropositive at baseline and went on to develop AIDS were selected from the larger cohort. Strikingly, 12 to 18 months prior to the development of AIDS, there was a rise in all measures of depression, with a mean increase in CES-D scores to 45% above baseline. These changes reached a plateau 6 months prior to establishment of an AIDS diagnosis. It is difficult to reconcile the results of these two studies without postulating higher drop-out rates of depressed subjects in the former study, but the MACS data may be more robust since they examine a larger number of more homogeneous subjects over a longer duration.

While early research emphasized the importance of pre-existing axis I diagnoses as the predominant risk factor for depression in HIV-positive homosexual/bisexual men, more recent studies have challenged this view in this and other populations. In one of the previously cited studies by Rabkin, the strongest correlate of distress was current HIV symptoms rather than lifetime history of major depression (4). Lyketsos performed a cross-sectional analysis of inner-city adults beginning primary care for HIV (11). Over half of the individuals screened with the BDI and the General Health Questionnaire (GHQ) had scores above the screening threshhold; comorbid substance abuse, lower level of education, and current unemployment all predicted higher levels of distress or higher screening scores, whereas the past psychiatric history was not significantly associated with either. In contrast, the association between depression and axis II diagnoses may have been underestimated in prior studies. Johnson found a 19% prevalence of personality disorders in a cohort of HIV-seropositive and HIV-seronegative homosexual men (12). The infected individuals had early, minimally symptomatic disease; those with personality disorders had higher levels of self-reported psychiatric symptoms and a six-fold increase in current axis I diagnoses, the majority of which were depression. Psychological factors have also emerged as risk factors. In a series of publications, Fukunishi and colleagues have examined the relationship between coping style and the presence of depressive symptoms in Japanese patients (13-15). Avoidance coping responses correlated with higher depression scores although none of their subjects met diagnostic criteria for a major depressive disorder. Furthermore, those with higher depression indices tended to have more somatic symptoms. Patients with HIV infection also had higher avoidance scores than individuals with either end-stage renal disease or breast cancer.

The latter point emphasizes recent observations about the social factors which appear to significantly contribute to depression in HIV-infected adults. Although there are confounding variables which exist, there are now some data from multiple geographic regions (including Thailand and Japan) that suggest that people residing in areas with recent introduction of HIV may be at particular risk for depressive symptoms (15,16). This raises the question of stigmatization and social isolation playing an important etiologic role in depression. In support of this notion are numerous reports that clearly document the correlation between depression score and lack of perceived social support (1,3,15,17,18). Current unemployment may also be an important co-factor (1).

Finally, questions about frequency of suicide and suicidality in HIV-seropositive patients have also been revisited. Occasional reports documenting increased prevalence continue to appear , but these tend to draw from selected populations already receiving psychiatric care (19). Two larger epidemiological studies have now addressed this issue and avoided this bias. Ndimbie examined over 800 homosexual or bisexual men who were enrolled in the Multicenter AIDS Cohort Study (MACS); 35% were HIV-infected (20). In the whole group, there were 5 unexpected deaths (2 in HIV-seropositive individuals), only one of which was classified by the coroner as a suicide. By comparison, 70 deaths were attributed to complications of HIV infection. The annual rate of 0.08% of otherwise unexpected deaths did not differ from the incidence in age and race matched controls. Dannenberg and colleagues carried out a prospective cohort study using the United States National Death Index to examine suicide rates in over 4000 HIV-infected military service applicants (21). These cases were matched with HIV-seronegative applicants who were disqualified from military service due to other medical conditions and followed for a median of 70 months. The relative risk of suicide in both cases and controls was increased by approximately two-fold compared to the general population, but there was no significant difference between the HIV-seropositive and HIV-seronegative applicants. While the former study may lack power because of the sample size, and the latter may underestimate suicide incidence due to an oversampling of individuals with early, asymptomatic HIV infection, together they do not support the magnitude of increased risk of suicide claimed by earlier reports (e.g. as much as a thirty-fold increase).

Pharmacotherapy of HIV-related Depression

There are no studies comparing the efficacy of a medication or class of antidepressant medications in depressed HIV-positive versus HIV-negative subjects. Thus, most inferences about efficacy in this setting versus other depressed populations must be drawn from historical data.

A variety of traditional and alternative antidepressant regimens have been examined. Rabkin performed a placebo-controlled trial with standard doses of imipramine in 97 HIV-seropositive depressed patients, approximately a third of whom had been diagnosed with AIDS (22). Over six weeks, there was a 20% dropout rate due to medication side effects. Using the Hamilton Depression Rating Scale (HAM-D) and Brief Symptom Inventory as the major outcome measures, subjects who completed the course of active drug had a 74% response rate, compared to a 26% response rate in the placebo group. Two recent studies suggest similar results with selective serotonin reuptake inhibitors (SSRI's). Grassi treated 15 patients with open label paroxetine at a daily dose of 20 mg (23). There was excellent tolerance of the medication, and all subjects had significant improvements of HAM-D scores, including the ten individuals with major depressive disorders. Ferrando enrolled 33 depressed men and women with symptomatic HIV disease into a six week open label study of 3 different SSRI's (paroxetine, fluoxetine, or sertraline) (24). Nine individuals dropped out within 3 weeks of beginning study medication because of adverse effects. Of the patients that completed the six week course of therapy, all experienced improvement in affective and somatic symptoms. Thus, experience with newer antidepressants has been consistent with findings from the initial trials of tricyclic antidepressants, with response rates of approximately 75% and a significant rate of discontinuation due to adverse effects. In the absence of studies which directly compare classes of agents, it is not possible to definitively say whether SSRI's are better tolerated by this population.

Other pharmacologic approaches for depression that have been studied include stimulants and anabolic steroids. Wagner conducted an open label trial of dextroamphetamine in 24 men who met DSM-III-R criteria for a depressive disorder and who also had significant complaints of low energy (25). All had CD4 cell counts of <200/mm^3. Eighteen of the nineteen men who completed six weeks of treatment (median daily dosage of 10 mg) had increased energy and improved mood. The same group also noted that testosterone replacement resulted in a response rate of 81% (26). The rationale for this approach is that a significant minority of HIV-infected men have been found to have mild decreases in levels of endogenous anabolic steroids. Again, the results of small open label trials must be taken cautiously, but these results do suggest that classes of agents other than the classic antidepressants may provide benefit in at least a subset of depressed, HIV-infected patients.

Psychological and Psychiatric Effects of the Improving Prognosis of HIV Infection

Over the past several years, as newer regimens of highly active antiretroviral therapy have increased in availability, dramatic changes in the health of infected people with access to these therapies have occurred. There has been a decline in the rate of AIDS cases and AIDS mortality, and these demographic changes have been reflected in decreasing inpatient censuses and less frequent outpatient visits for complications of HIV disease. Potent antiretroviral therapy has allowed some previously disabled individuals with advanced HIV disease to resume many of their pre-morbid activities and even to return to the work force. Yet despite all of this optimistic news, the psychological effects upon individuals with HIV disease may be complex. For some, the chance of receiving state of the art medical treatment may be diminished by poverty, homelessness, or other barriers to care. Others may experience guilt of having options available to them that were not available to family, loved ones, or friends who succumbed to HIV disease. Many people have described the profound adjustment of resetting expectations from a terminal illness to a chronic treatable disease, and patients who have benefitted from newer drug regimens wonder about the long term duration of these effects. All of this makes the ultimate impact of these medical advances on psychiatric issues a matter of speculation. It is clear that previous research in this arena does not predict what will happen in this new era of medical therapy, and one hopes that future efforts will be refined on the basis of the enormous amount of work that has preceded them.

References

1. Katz MH, Douglas JM, Bolan GA, et al. Depression and use of mental health services among HIV-infected men. AIDS Care, 1996, 8:433-42.
2. Judd FK, Mijch AM. Depressive symptoms in patients with HIV infection. Aust New Zeal J Psych, 1996, 30:104-9.
3. Perkins DO, Stern RA, Golden RN, et al. Mood disorders in HIV infection: prevalence and risk factors in a nonepicenter of the AIDS epidemic. Am J Psych, 1994, 151:233-6.
4. Rabkin JG, Ferrando SJ, Jacobsberg LB, Fishman B. Prevalence of axis I disorders in an AIDS cohort: a cross-sectional, controlled study. Comp Psych, 1997, 38:146-54.
5. Lipsitz JD, Williams JB, Rabkin JG, et al. Psychopathology in male and female intravenous drug user with and without HIV infection. Am J Psych, 1994, 151:1662-8.
6. Maj M, Janssen R, Starace F, et al. WHO neuropsychiatric AIDS study, cross-sectional phase I. Study design and psychiatric findings. Arch Gen Psych, 1994, 51:39-49.
7. Perkins DO, Lesserman J, Stern RA, et al. Somatic symptoms and HIV infection: relationship to depressive symptoms and indicators of HIV disease. Am J Psych, 1995, 152:1776-81.
8. O'Dell MW, Meighen M, Riggs RV. Correlates of fatigue in HIV infection prior to AIDS: a pilot study. Disability Rehab, 1996, 18:249-54.
9. Rabkin JG, Goetz RR, Remien RH, et al. Stability of mood despite HIV illness progression in a group of homosexual men. Am J Psych, 1997, 154:231-8.
10. Lyketsos CG, Hoover DR, Guccione M, et al. Changes in depressive symptoms as AIDS develops. The Multicenter AIDS Cohort Study. Am J Psych, 1996, 153:1430-7.
11. Lyketsos CG, Hutton H, Fishman M, Schwartz J, Treisman GJ. Psychiatric morbidity on entry to an HIV primary care clinic. AIDS, 1996, 10:1033-9.
12. Johnson JG, Williams JB, Rabkin JG, Goetz RR, Remien RH. Axis I psychiatric symptoms associated with HIV infection and personality disorder. Am J Psych, 1995, 152:551-4.
13. Fukunishi I, Hosaka T, Negishi M, et al. Subclinical depressive symptoms in HIV are related to avoidance coping responses: a comparison with end-stage renal failure and breast cancer. Psych Reports, 1996, 78:483-8.
14. Fukunishi I, Hayashi M, Matsumoto T, et al. Liaison psychiatry and HIV infection (1): avoidance coping responses associated with depressive symptoms accompanying somatic complaints. Psych and Clin Neurosciences, 1997, 51:1-4.

15. Fukunishi I, Hosaka T, Negishi M, et al. Avoidance coping behaviors and low social support are related to depressive symptoms in HIV-positive patients in Japan. Psychosomatics, 1997, 38:113-8.
16. Maj M. Depressive syndromes and symptoms in subjects with human immunodeficiency virus (HIV) infection. Br J Psych, 1996, Suppl:117-22.
17. McClure JB, Catz SL, Prejean J, Brantley PJ, Jones GN. Factors associated with depression in a heterogeneous HIV-infected sample. J Psychosomatic Res, 1996, 40:407-15.
18. Rosenfeld B, Breitbart W, McDonald MV, et al. Pain in ambulatory AIDS patients. II. Impact of pain on psychological functioning and quality of life. Pain, 1996, 68:323-8.
19. O'Dowd MA, Biderman DJ, McKegney FP. Incidence of suicidality in AIDS and HIV-positive patients attending a psychiatry outpatient program. Psychosomatics, 1993, 34:33-40.
20. Ndimbie OK, Perper JA, Kingsley L, Harty L, Winkelstein A. Sudden unexpected death in a male homosexual cohort. Am J Forensic Med Path, 1994, 15:247-50.
21. Dannenberg AL, McNeil JG, Brundage JF, Brookmeyer R. Suicide and HIV infection. Mortality follow-up of 4147 HIV-seropositive military service recruits. JAMA, 1996, 276:1743-6.
22. Rabkin JG, Rabkin R, Harrison W, Wagner G. Effect of imipramine on mood and enumerative measures of immune status in depressed patinets with HIV illness. Am J Psych, 1994, 151:516-23.
23. Grassi B, Gambini O, Garghentini G, Lazzarin A, Scarone S. Efficacy of paroxetine for the treatment of depression in the context of HIV infection. Pharmacopsych, 1997, 30:70-1.
24. Ferrando SJ, Goldman JD, Charness WE. Selective serotonin reuptake inhibitor treatment of depression in symptomatic HIV infection and AIDS. Improvements in affective and somatic symptoms. Gen Hosp Psych, 1997, 19:89-97.
25. Wagner GJ, Rabkin JG, Rabkin R. Dextroamphetamine as a treatment for depression and low enegy in AIDS patients: a pilot study. J Psychosom Res, 1997, 42:407-11.
26. Wagner GJ, Rabkin JG, Rabkin R. A comparative analysis of standard and alternative antidepressants in the treatment of human immunodeficiency virus patients. Comp Psych, 1996, 37:402-8.

Euthanasia, Social Policy and Empirical Data

Harvey Max Chochinov MD, Ph.D. FRCPC, Professor of Psychiatry, University of Manitoba, Soros Faculty Scholar, Project on Death in America, PZ202 - 771 Bannatyne Avenue, Winnipeg, Manitoba, Canada R3E 0T4

SUMMARY: Many opinions have been expressed about the issue of euthanasia and physician assisted suicide. These opinions tend to be passionate and highly polarized. Largely absent from these discussions is the issue of empirical data, pertaining to our understanding of patients who might make death-hastening requests.

This chapter reviews the small but growing literature which derives from data based sources. This data examines a number of issues that are salient to the euthanasia -physician assisted suicide debate. Included within this review are the following: 1) an overview of social policies regarding euthanasia/ physician assisted suicide in various different constituencies, 2) studies examining physician attitudes and practices, 3) public perceptions, and determinants of endorsement, of death hastening practices, 4) patient mediated variables - including mental health considerations - influencing a patients desire for hastened death. Such information provides a less impassioned understanding of these issues, and may help inform the development of social policy, research priorities and clinical standards of palliative care.

Key Words: Euthanasia, Physician assisted suicide, empirical data

The debate regarding euthanasia and physician assisted suicide has largely revolved around rhetoric, anecdote, and passion. Conspicuously absent from this dialogue has been the 'voice' of empirical data pertaining to patients who might request the hastening of their death in anticipation of a foreshortened life expectancy. In spite this paucity of data, the debate undauntedly wages on at an unprecedented pace. In Canada this has included a formal review of these issues by a Special Senate Committee, appointed in order to conduct public hearings to determine the extent to which these practices are to be condoned, endorsed, and even possibly decriminalized.

There is a small but growing literature that provides some insight into the mental and physical status of patients making death-hastening decisions. The extent to which this kind of information can - or even should - guide social policy is a matter of some contention. Ethicists such as Pellegrino argue that empirical data is of limited value in guiding ethical decisions that pertain to the resolution of moral questions [1]. There is, however, no debate that such data can help inform our understanding of dying patients and their end of life decision making processes. As a special case of suicide, one might also argue that mental health considerations are of fundamental concern in any thorough review of these issues. The extent to which physical and psychiatric morbidity can be understood as risk factors in death hastening decisions -and the degree to which this can inform or guide social policy - is the focus of this report. Using definitions outlined by Sawyer et al [2], "euthanasia" refers to positive acts of commission, such as lethal injections, undertaken deliberately by physicians to end the lives of patients who have explicitly requested to die. "Assisted suicide" refers to the provision of advice or the means for an individual to commit suicide.

Current Canadian Social Policy

The current laws in Canada prohibiting euthanasia and physician assisted suicide fall within the jurisdiction of the Federal criminal code. Euthanasia is essentially regarded as an act of murder, while assisted suicide is covered under Section 241 of the code. While attempting suicide was decriminalized in 1972, aiding or abetting suicide remains a punishable offense by up to 14 years imprisonment [3].

The strongest challenge to Section 241 came by way of the case, Rodriguez vs. British Columbia. At the age of 42, Sue Rodriguez - a woman with amyotrophic lateral sclerosis - took her request to have physician-assisted suicide available at a time of her choosing all the way to the Supreme Court of Canada. She argued that the law against assisted suicide was in violation of the Canadian Charter of Rights and Freedoms, on the grounds that section 15 of the Charter provides for equal treatment under the law for people with physical disabilities. While able bodied persons have the capacity to take their own lives without criminal liability, Ms Rodriguez argued that the law is discriminatory because it places disabled persons at risk of prosecution in seeking assistance to commit suicide. In a decidedly spit decision (5 to 4) the Court ruled against Ms Rodriguez, arguing that it is indeed reasonable that some patients must endure physical and emotional suffering in order to maintain the sanctity of life and to protect vulnerable individuals from the risk of involuntary termination of their lives. In spite of the Courts' decision, Ms Rodriguez did take her own life with the assistance of an anonymous physician.

Shortly after the death of Sue Rodriguez, the Canadian Government established a Special Senate Committee of Euthanasia and Assisted Suicide. This committee heard from hundreds of witnesses across the country and submitted their final report in June, 1995 [4].   Although they ultimately recommended that section 241 of the criminal code not be amended and that euthanasia should remain a criminal offense, they were decidedly split in rendering their decision   (the chairperson, Senator Joan Neiman, has been very vocal in her support of the minority opinion). They also recommended that in cases of euthanasia undertaken with essentially merciful intent, a new category of murder, or "compassionate homicide", should be incorporated into the code and carry with it a less severe penalty [4]. Given the divisive nature of the Senates' recommendations, and social policy decisions being made in other jurisdictions regarding these issues, the ultimate direction of Canadian social policy on euthanasia and physician assisted suicide remains far from certain.

Euthanasia and Assisted Suicide in other Jurisdictions

The issue of euthanasia and assisted suicide has received unprecedented recent attention in the United States.   This has largely followed in the wake of highly publicized disclosures by physicians who have participated in these practices [5,6]. The activities of Dr. Jack Kevorkian, a retired Michigan pathologist and his "suicide machine", have also focused the attention of the American public on the alleged right of consenting dying patients to receive assistance in hastening their death   [7]. While such practices remain illegal in most states, Dr. Kevorkian has nevertheless been acquitted by the Michigan courts of any wrongdoing for his role in assisting suicides.

A number of states, including Washington in 1991 and California in 1992, have held public ballots to decriminalize euthanasia and assisted suicide.   Although both these proposals were defeated, Oregon voters approved a limited proposal to permit physician assisted suicide, but not euthanasia [8]. Measure 16 in Oregon was directed at competent, terminally ill patients with a life expectancy of less than six months (as determined by two physicians).   The patient is required to make the request at least three times within 15 days, with the final request in writing.   Provisions are to be made for counseling should the physician believe there are psychiatric factors influencing the patient's decision. The implementation of Measure 16 was blocked by a federal court judge on the day it was to become law.   Both the National

Right to Life Committee and the Americas with Disabilities Act [9,10] have contended that it violates constitutional guarantees of equal protection and due process.

Without a doubt, the most profound event impacting the American euthanasia debate has been the recent U.S. Supreme Court's review of the Ninth and Second Circuit Court decisions, wherein state laws banning assisted suicide were overturned. Both lower court decisions concluded that state laws banning assistance in suicide were unconstitutional as applied to doctors and their dying patients [11]. The wording of the Second Circuit Court opinion indicated that the state "has no interest in prolonging a life that is ending" [12]. It has been suggested that this should serve as a "chilling reminder of the low priority given to the dying when it comes to state resources and protection" [13]. In a unanimous decision, the Supreme Court recently ruled that there is no constitutional right to physician-assisted suicide.

On May 25, 1995, the parliament of Australia's Northern Territory passed the Northern Territory Rights of the Terminally Ill Act, containing most of the procedural safeguards as Oregon's Measure 16, but legalizing voluntary euthanasia. This law was enacted in July 1996. It stipulated that patients must be deemed to have a life expectancy of less than 12 months, be competent, and the decision to end their life have been made freely, voluntarily and after due consideration. Psychiatric consultation must also take place as part of the evaluative process, confirming that the patient does not have a "treatable clinical depression" [14]. While this legislation enabled four Northern Territories patients to receive physician assistance in hastening their death, the policy was overturned by the Australian Senate.

Undoubtedly, the jurisdiction with the most experience in its social policies regarding physician-hastened death is the Netherlands. Euthanasia and assisted suicide are still technically illegal in Holland (punishable by up to 12 years and 3 years respectively). However, physicians who assist patients in hastening their death have not been subject to prosecution since 1984, provided they do so within specified guidelines. These include that the patient is competent, the request is freely initiated and persistent over time; the patient's physical or mental suffering is unbearable; all treatment alternatives have been exhausted or refused; a second consulting physician concurs with the euthanasia decision; the circumstances surrounding the patient's death are carefully documented [15]. Today, most Dutch physicians consider euthanasia and physician assisted suicide components of compassionate medical practice.

Empirical Data

Public Perceptions:

There is relativity little empirically derived data which helps inform our understanding of social policies vis-à-vis euthanasia and physician assisted suicide. Much of the existing data consists of population based surveys, examining attitudes toward physician hastened death. One of the earliest such surveys took place in 1950, and reported that 36 percent of American adults favored the legalization of euthanasia for patients with advanced terminal illness [16]. Since then, public support for this type of legislative reform has been steadily increasing. A recent study by Genuis et al [17] reported that 65 percent of a random sample of Edmonton residents were in favor of legalizing euthanasia for the terminally ill.

Several demographic characteristics have been found to be associated with attitudes towards euthanasia. For example, level of endorsement appears to vary by racial group with whites being consistently more in favor than African-Americans (by a margin of about 20 percent) [16]. It would also appear that younger respondents express stronger endorsement than those over age 50 years. One might speculate that such data implies a waning of support for euthanasia and physician assisted suicide as the reality of ones own death approaches. Data from patient cohort studies (see *Patient Attitudes*) lend additional support for this interpretation.

Physician Attitudes:

In a recent review of studies addressing physician attitudes towards euthanasia [18], the level of support ranged from 35 percent to 60 percent. If legalized, 25 percent to 50 percent of physicians reported their willingness to practice it. A study by Kinsella and Verhoef [19] in Alberta found that of 1391 physicians polled, 51% felt the law should be changed to permit euthanasia, while only 28 percent indicated a willingness to actually participate. A more recent study in Alberta found that 60-80% of physicians opposed legalization of euthanasia and assisted suicide, while 50-60% of the public and terminally ill patients agreed with it [20].

A number of recent publications have further clarified the extent to which physicians would support legislative reform and /or participate in actual death hastening practices. A study by Back et al [21] reported an anonymous mail survey, answered by a total of 828 physicians. Within the prior year, 12 percent of responding physicians reported having received one or more explicit requests for physician assisted suicide, and 4 percent received one or more requests for euthanasia. Of 156 patients who had requested physician assisted suicide, 38 (24%) received prescriptions, 21 of whom died as a result. Of 58 patients requesting euthanasia, 14 (24%) received parenteral medication and died. Of note, physicians involved in these decisions rarely sought out consultation from their medical (15%) or psychiatric (24%) colleagues. Furthermore, these physicians reported primarily non-physical (i.e. psychological) sources of symptom distress as having led their patients to seek out death hastening measures.

A recent study by Lee et al examined the views of physicians in Oregon towards the prospect of legalizing assisted suicide [22]. They conducted a cross sectional mail survey of all physicians who would be eligible to prescribe lethal medication in the event that the Oregon law is upheld. Of the 2761 respondents (70 percent response rate), 60 percent thought physician assisted suicide should be legal in some cases; 46 percent indicated a willingness to prescribe lethal doses of medication if it were legal to do so. Twenty-one percent of respondents indicated having previously received requests for assisted suicide, with 7 percent having complied. It is noteworthy that half the respondents in this study were not confident they could predict that a patient had less than six months to live (a critical survival threshold beyond which, according to the Oregon Death with Dignity Act, patients would not be deemed eligible for physician assisted suicide). One third of respondents also reported not being confidence they could recognize depression in a patient asking for a lethal dose of medication.

A fascinating study by Emanuel et al compared the attitudes of oncology patients, oncologists and the general public regarding euthanasia and physician assisted suicide [23]. Consistent with prior reports, physicians were found to be less favorably disposed toward euthanasia and assisted suicide than either patients or the public at large (22.7/45.5% verses 68.2/70.5% verses 65.6/ 66.5% respectively in response to an "unremitting pain" vignette). In a multivariate logistic regression analysis, patients in pain were significantly more likely to find euthanasia and physician assisted suicide unacceptable (odds ratio 2.3 [95% CI 1.0-5.3]). Patients over the age of 50 years were also significantly more likely to find euthanasia and physician assisted suicide unacceptable (p<0.5). As has been consistently reported in other studies of this kind (17,20), religiosity was found to be highly correlated with non-endorsement of death hastening practices. Finding physician assisted suicide unacceptable, given religiosity, was OR= 3.5 [2.2-5.6] amongst oncologists, 2.8 [1.4-6.3] for oncology patients and 4.3 [2.1-8.8] for the general public. Patients with depression were significantly more likely to feel that discussions which explicitly included mention of euthanasia or physician assisted suicide would increase trust in their physician (6.9[2.0-23.6]); interesting, patients with pain believed these same discussions would not increase trust (0.3-[0.1-0.8]). Patients with substantial pain or whose cancer had relapsed were significantly more likely to say they would change their oncologist if told he or she "had provided euthanasia or assisted suicide" for other patients (12.3 [1.6-94.6] and 4.0 [1.3-12.1], respectively). Such data strongly suggests that endorsement of these measures diminishes as the reality of ones death invariably approaches.

While most studies addressing the issue of euthanasia and physician assisted suicide have done so in the context of cancer populations, a recent study by Lee et al examined physician attitudes and practices amongst patients with human-immunodeficiency virus disease [24]. Using an anonymous, self administered questionnaire, these authors surveyed all 228 physicians in the Community Consortium providing health care to patients infected with HIV in the San Francisco Bay area. Of the one hundred eighteen questionnaires evaluated, respondents reported a mean of 7.9 "direct" and 13.7 "indirect" requests from patients for death hastening assistance. Forty-eight percent of physicians said they would likely grant the request of a patient with AIDS for assistance in a suicide (compared with 28 percent of respondents in a similar 1990 survey). Estimating the number of times they had acquiesced to such requests, 53 percent said they had done so at least once (mean of 4.2; median,1.0; range,0-100). A multivariate analysis, examining variables associated with physicians having assisted in a suicide, found the following emerged as significant; having a higher number of patients with AIDS who had died (OR 1.36 CI 1.25-2.4 p=0.02); having received a higher number of indirect requests from patients for death hastening assistance (1.08 [1.01-1.11] p=0.03); the physician having a stated gay, lesbian, or bisexual orientation (2.99 [1.07-8.30] p=0.04); and having a higher "intention to assist" score, as determined from physician responses to a case vignette (1.93 [1.25- 2.40] p=0.001). It would thus seem that physicians' decision to participate in death hastening practices is substantially influenced by a variety of highly personal characteristics.

It appears that physicians from different medical specialties have different opinions about euthanasia. Those practicing in areas most highly exposed to dying patients (e.g. oncologists, hematologists) have been found to have the least favorable attitudes [25,26], while psychiatrist are apparently most favorably inclined [26]. A study by Ganzini et al [26] examined the attitudes of Oregon psychiatrist toward physician assisted suicide. An anonymous questionnaire was answered by 321 psychiatrist (77 percent response rate), 69 percent of whom felt that physician assisted suicide may be morally acceptable under some circumstances. Fifty- six percent of respondents favored implementation of Measure 16. Psychiatrists opposed to Measure 16 were much more likely to refuse performing a psychiatric evaluation (to determine whether or not a psychiatric disorder was impairing the judgment of a patient requesting assisted suicide) than those in favor (28% verses 68%, respectively; c2=61.3,d.f.=3,p<0.0001). When asked to rate their level of confidence in determining (with a single evaluation) whether a psychiatric disorder might be impairing the judgment of a patient requesting assisted suicide, 51 percent were not at all confidence, 43 percent were somewhat confident, and only six percent were very confident. Particularly fascinating, those who favored Measure 16 were significantly more confident in their ability to adequately assess the patient in the context of a single evaluation compared to those who opposed it ($\chi2$=28.1,df=2,p<0.0001). It would thus appear that ones political position on euthanasia and assisted suicide might correlate highly with ones perceived clinical acumen in evaluating patients death hastening requests.

Patient Attitudes:

The level of public support for euthanasia and physician assisted suicide would lead one to suspect that, amongst the ill or dying, endorsement would be overwhelming. Indeed, a study of interest in physician assisted suicide among ambulatory HIV-infected patients (N=378) reported that 63 percent supported policies favoring physician assisted suicide, and 55 percent acknowledged having considered physician assisted suicide as an option for themselves [27]. As reported in other studies [23,28], level of depressive symptomatology was found to be highly correlated with interest in physician assisted suicide (t=2.68,df=374,p=0.008). However, these authors did not investigate dying patients requesting physician assisted suicide but rather, asked ambulatory patients with HIV / AIDS about their interest in physician assisted suicide.

Perhaps the most compelling data regarding the extent to which patients actually partake of death hastening measures comes from the Netherlands. In January 1990, Professor J. Remmelink, Attorney General of the Dutch Supreme Court, commissioned a nationwide study to determine the extent to which euthanasia and other medical decisions concerning the end of life were taking place in Holland. Three studies by van der Mass et al were undertaken, including detailed interviews with 405 physicians, the mailing of questionnaires to the physicians of a sample of 7000 deceased persons, and collecting information about 2250 deaths using a prospective survey among the respondents to the interviews [29]. The cumulative data from these studies determined that euthanasia accounts for 1.8 percent of all deaths in Holland; assisted suicide accounts for 0.3 percent of all deaths (together, corresponding to approximately 1990 deaths). It appears that 25,000 patients per year ask assurance from their doctors that they will assist them if their suffering becomes unbearable. Nearly nine thousand explicit requests are received yearly, of which less than one third are agreed to. The majority (68 percent) of those patients whose requests are subsequently granted appear to have had cancer. A rather disturbing finding was evidence suggesting that 0.8 percent of deaths resulted from life-terminating acts wherein an explicit and persistent request had not been made. While the authors suggest that in nearly all circumstances, these measures were undertaken with compassionate intent, others have argued that this represents evidence of a "slippery slope"[30].

These studies also attempted to have physicians reconstruct why they believe their patients sought out death hastening measures. Loss of dignity was mentioned in 57% of cases, pain in 46 percent, unworthy dying (46 percent), being dependent on others (33 percent), or tiredness of life (23 percent); pain alone was cited as a reason in less than one percent of cases. The prominence of psychological and existential concerns, over and above physical distress, is particularly interesting. Such data is, however, essentially post hoc and anecdotal. As such, it provides limited insight into why patients sought out death hastening measures.

van der Maas et al recently published a follow-up report [31], documenting the extent to which euthanasia and physician assisted suicide practices have evolved since 1990. They conducted two studies in 1995, the first involving interviews with 405 physicians and the second involving questionnaires mailed to physicians who had attended 6060 deaths as identified from death certificates. The former study found that euthanasia and physician assisted suicide accounted for 2.3 percent and 0.4 percent of all deaths respectively. The death certificate study reported similar findings, with euthanasia and physician assisted suicide accounting for 2.4 percent and 0.2 percent of all deaths respectively. The number of requests for euthanasia or assisted suicide increased from 25,100 in 1990, to 34,500 in 1995;the number of explicit requests increased from 8,000 in 1990 to 9,700 in 1995. As in their 1990 study [29], a small percentage of cases (i.e. 0.7 percent) were reported wherein life had been ended without the explicit, concurrent request of the patient. These authors conclude that there is no evidence to suggest that decision making has become less careful. However one reads their data, what is abundantly clear is that only a small minority of dying patients - small when one considers the level of endorsement expressed amongst the general public - actually partake of these death hastening measures. This raises the distinct possibility that people are extremely poor at making accurate predictions about their end of life decision preferences from a vantage point of health.

What happens to decisions regarding death-hastening processes as the reality of death approaches? An Australian study [32] approached this question, using an epidemiological survey of people aged 70 or more live. Participants were asked whether they had repeatedly felt they wanted to die within the last two weeks. Of the 923 elderly respondents, only 21 reported repeatedly having had a wish to die during the previous two weeks. Factors associated with the wish to die included: aged 80+ (OR 2.0, [95% CI 0.8-4.8]); female (1.7[0.7-4.2]); not married (2.9 [1.1-7.6]); depressive disorder (14.6 [5.2-41.0]); cognitive impairment (3.3 [1.2-9.3]); poor self-rated health (12.7[4.7-34.3]); disabled (5.9[2.1-16.4]); in pain (5.2[2.2-13.9]); hearing impaired (5.6 [2.3-13.9]); visually impaired (14.6 [5.7-37.3]); in residential care (17.3[7.0-42.9]). A study by Seale and Addington-Hall [33] approached this very question using the results of two surveys in England of relatives and others who had known people in samples drawn from death certificates. They reported on a sample of 3696 people dying in 1990 and an earlier national sample of 639 people who had died in 1987. These authors found that, according to respondent reports, 3.6% of the deceased had asked for euthanasia at some point in their last year of life. A logistic regression model of 'cancer patient interest in dying earlier' and 'reported requests for euthanasia' found that pain, loss of control, mental impairment, and dependency entered as highly significant (p<0.01)(pain was not found to be significant in the non cancer logistic regression model). Social class and religiosity were largely found to be insignificant in influencing preferences regarding an early death or request for euthanasia.

In a study of one hundred cancer patients [34], Owen et al conducted interviews to determine their attitudes towards a range of final life events. Patients who expressed a desire for death to hasten were significantly less likely to be married (p<0.5). They rated significantly higher on measures of hopelessness (12.3 SD 4 vs. 8 SD 0.3 p<0.001), anxiety (6.3 SD 4 vs. 3.9 SD 3 p<0.05) and depression (6.3 SD 4 vs. 2.8 SD 3 p<0.001). A logistic regression model confirmed that lack of social support and hopelessness were independent predictors of a current wish for death to hasten, accounting for 40 percent of the variance. Such data, obtained from actual patient populations, begins to suggest that a desire for death may derive from potentially remediable sources of symptom distress.

Mental Health Considerations:

A study by Brown et al [35] was one of the first to critically evaluated a desire for death amongst the terminally ill. They reported that 10 of 44 patients in a palliative care facility endorsed a desire for hastened death. Of those 10 patients, all were reported as having concomitant clinical depression. Since than, other studies [36] have helped established the prevalence of major depression amongst the terminally ill to be in the order of 9-13 percent (depending on which diagnostic system was used and the level of stringency set in determining case identification). Depression is a critical consideration in discussions of cancer suicide, given that it is thought to place patients at up to 25 times the risk of completed suicide compared to the general population [37].

Depression has also been found to be important in terms of patient preferences for life sustaining medical therapy. Ganzini et al [38] found that among elderly depressed patients, a clinically significant increase in desire for life sustaining medical therapies followed treatment of those subjects who had initially been most severely depressed. These patients were also found to have initially been more hopeless, and more likely to overestimate the risks and underestimate the benefits of treatment. They suggested that decisions about life sustaining therapy, especially amongst the severely depressed, should be discouraged until after treatment of their depression. Similar findings were reported by Hooper et al [39]. They examined 22 elderly patients referred to a Psychogeriatric Service with major depression. They found that moderate or severe depression in this patient population was associated with a high degree of refusal of life sustained treatments (as measured by responses to hypothetical acute life threatening illness scenarios). Treatment of depression led to an increased acceptance of these therapeutic interventions.

A study of 200 terminally ill patients, recruited from a palliative care facility, reported that 44.5 percent acknowledged at least a fleeting desire for an early death [28]. In most instances these episodes were brief and did not reflect a sustained or committed desire as would be required in a death hastening decision. However, 8.5 percent of the study group (17 patients) reported a persistent, genuine desire for an early death. The prevalence of clinical depression in this group was significantly higher than amongst patients without a desire for death (58.8% verses 7.7%;chi^2=33.66,df=1,p<0.001;OR=17.1, 95% CI=5.0-60.0). The prevalence of pain which was of moderate severity or greater was higher amongst patients with a desire for death (76.5%) compared to patients without a desire for death (46.2%);chi^2=4.57,df=1,p=0.03;OR=3.8[1.1-14.4]). Perceived level of social support was lower in the former group (66.1 mm [VAS scale]) compared with the latter (85.0 mm) (t=2.57,df=197,p=0.01). To investigate the conjoint predictive value of those variables which emerged as significant in the univariate analyses (i.e. depression, pain, and a low level of social support), a stepwise multiple logistic regression analysis was conducted. Depression entered as the only significant predictor of group classification (F=23.33,df=1,193,p<0.001). Scores on the Beck Depression Inventory [40] showed significant collinearity with ratings of pain (r=0.33,N=196,p<0.001) and family support (r=-0.25,N=196,p<0.001). As a result, the other two measures did not make a unique contribution to the regression model once the effect of depression had been removed. The importance of depression is further underscored by an Australian study, in which the current preferences for euthanasia were examined in a sample of elderly depressed patients [41]. Of eighteen patients whose depression subsequently improved with treatment, eight (44%) indicated an initial wish for someone else to end their life. After treatment, only two (11%) maintained their original position, with six (75%) having essentially changed their minds.

The study by Chochinov et al [28] also attempted to address the question of temporal stability of desire for death in this patient population. Of the 17 patients who had originally endorsed a desire for hastened death, only six were available to be re-interviewed two weeks later. The others had either died, become too ill to participate, or had opted for discharge to home care. Of these six patients, four demonstrated a decline in their desire for death to the extent that they no longer scored above our operational cutoff for defining a serious and pervasive desire (4 on the desire for death rating scale). This finding is all the more poignant when one considers that, in Holland, it has been reported that 65 percent of all euthanasia deaths occur within two weeks of the initial request [42].

A further attempt to examine the temporal stability of ' will to live' took place in a study of 167 end stage hospitalized cancer patients receiving palliative care [43]. Each patient's will to live was measured with a self report 100mm visual analog scale. A similar approach was used to quantify other sources of symptom distress including pain, nausea, shortness of breath, appetite, drowsiness; depression, sense of well being, anxiety and activity. All measures were obtained twice daily throughout the course of each patient's hospitalization. Maximal fluctuations in 'will to live' were examined over various time intervals (12hrs, 24hrs; 1, 2, 3 and 4 weeks). Fifty percent of patients demonstrated a fluctuation of 40 to 100mm on the 'will to live' visual analog scale within a 12 hour time frame; at the 4 week interval, this fluctuation ranged between 80 and 100mm. A series of stepwise regressions of all symptom variables on 'will to live' were carried out at the time of admission, 24 hours later;1,2,3 and 4 weeks. These models accounted for between 20% and 43% of the variance (p<0.5). The four main predictor variables (all sharing considerable covariance) were depression, anxiety, shortness of breath and sense of well being. While the latter was a strong predictor in all models, the prominence of the other variables shifted over time. These findings would suggest that amongst dying patients, 'will to live' is a highly unstable construct whose determinants shift as death approaches.

Final Thoughts

While empirical data may not offer the definitive word in helping guide social policies pertaining to moral issues, it does nevertheless provide compelling information. In determining policy decisions regarding euthanasia and physician assisted suicide, it is critical that we clearly understand the extent to which these practices are likely to be used and by whom. If incidence estimates from Holland [27,29] are placed in a Canadian context, one might anticipate 5,000 to 7,000 deaths a year resulting directly from physician involvement in death hastening measures. The data clearly suggests that the level of physical and psychological distress amongst these patients would be considerable. In many instances, this distress - possibly underlying a request for physician hastened death - would derive from remediable sources of suffering.

Although it is tempting to see social policy emanate from the will of a vocal majority, it is noteworthy that endorsement of euthanasia and physician assisted suicide may be inversely proportional to ones proximity to dying. Perhaps more critical attention must be focused on those whose fate and poor health have placed them closest to an impending death. Empirically based research emanating from this vantage point offers the potential to enhance palliative care, and the range of treatment options available, for patients nearing the end of life.

References

1. Pellegrino ED. The limitation of empirical research in ethics. J Clin Ethics 1995;6:149-151.
2. Sawyer DM, Williams JR, Lowy F. Canadian physicians and euthanasia: 2. Definitions and distinctions. Can Med Assoc J 1993;148:1463-1466.
3. Dickens BM. When terminally ill patients request death: assisted suicide before Canadian courts. J Palliative Care 1994;10:52-56.
4. Report of the Special Senate Committee on Euthanasia and Assisted Suicide. Ottawa: Senate of Canada (Cat. No. YC2-351/1-01E); 1995.
5. It's over Debbie. J Am Med Assoc 1988;258:272.
6. Quill TE. Death and dignity: a case of individualized decision making. N Engl J Med 1991;324:691-694.
7. Roberts J, Kjellstrand C. Jack Kevorkian: a medical hero. Br Med J 1996;312:1434.
8. Annas GJ. Death by prescription: the Oregon initiative. N Engl J Med 1994;331:1240-1243.
9. Kaufert JM. 'Euthanasia policy: disabled consumers' perspectives.' In: Sneiderman B, Kaufert JM (eds.), Euthanasia in the Netherlands: a model for Canada? Legal Research Institute of the University of Manitoba, 1994;55-68.
10. International League of Societies for Persons with Mental Handicap (ILSMH). Open Discussion Forum on New Bio-Ethical Issues. Budapest, Hungary 1991.
11. Annas GJ. The promised end - constitutional aspects of physician-assisted suicide. New Engl J Med 1996;335:683-687.
12. Minor, Quill v. Vacco 80. F.3d 716, 2nd Cir., 1996.
13. Foley KM. Competent care for the dying instead of physician-assisted suicide. N Engl J Med 1997;336:54-58.
14. Ryan CJ, Kaye M. Euthanasia in Australia - the northern territory rights of the terminally ill act. N Engl J Med 1996;334:326-328.
15. Mullens A. The Dutch experience with euthanasia: lessons for Canada? Can Med Assoc J 1995;152:1845-1852.
16. Blendon RJ, Szalay VS, Knox RA. Should physicians aid their patients in dying? The public perspective. J Am Med Assoc 1992;267:2658-2662.
17. Genuis SJ, Genuis SK, Chang V-C. Public attitudes toward the right to die. Can Med Assoc J 1994;150:701-708.
18. Chochinov HM, Wilson KG. The euthanasia debate: attitudes, practices and psychiatric considerations. Can J Psychiatry 1995;40:593-602.
19. Kinsella TD, Verhoef MJ. Alberta euthanasia survey: I. Physicians' opinions about the morality and legalization of active euthanasia. Can Med Assoc J 1993;148:1921-1926.
20. Suarez-Almazor ME, Belzile M, Bruera E. Euthanasia and physician-assisted suicide: a comparative survey of physicians, terminally ill cancer patients, and the general population. J Clin Oncology 1997;15:418-427.
21. Back AL, Wallace JI, Starks HE, et al. Physician-assisted suicide and euthanasia in Washington State. J Am Med Assoc 1996;275:919-925.

22. Lee MA, Nelson HD, Tilden VP, et al.   Legalizing assisted suicide - views of physicians in Oregon. N Engl J Med 1996;334:310-315.
23. Emanuel EJ, Fairclough DL, Daniels ER, et al.   Euthanasia and physician-assisted suicide: attitudes and experiences of oncology patients, oncologists, and the public.   Lancet 1996;347:1805-1810.
24. Slome, LR, Mitchell TF, Charlebois E, et al.   Physician-assisted suicide and patients with human immunodeficiency virus disease.   N Engl J Med 1997;336:417-421.
25. Cohen JS, Fihn SD, Boyko EJ, et al.   Attitudes toward assisted suicide and euthanasia among physicians in Washington State.   N Engl J Med 1994;331:89-94.
26. Ganzini L, Fenn DS, Lee MA, et al.   Attitudes of Oregon psychiatrists toward physician-assisted suicide.   Am J Psychiatry 1996;153:1469-1475.
27. Breitbart W, Rosenfeld BD, Passik SD.   Interest in physician-assisted suicide among ambulatory HIV-infected patients.   Am J Psychiatry 1996;153:238-242.
28. Chochinov HM, Wilson KG, Enns M, et al.   Desire for death in the terminally ill.   Am J Psychiatry 1995;152:1185-1191.
29. van der Maas PJ, van Delden JJM, Pijnenborg L, et al.   Euthanasia and other medical decisions concerning the end of life.   Lancet, 1991;338:669-674.
30. Angell M.   Euthanasia in the Netherlands - good news or bad?   N Engl J Med 1996;335:1676-1678.
31. van der Maas PJ, van der Wal G, Haverkate I, et al.   Euthanasia, physician-assisted suicide, and other medical practices involving the end of life in the Netherlands, 1990-1995.   N Engl J Med 1996;335:1699-1705.
32. Jorm AF, Henderson AS, Scott R, et al.   Factors associated with the wish to die in elderly people. Age Ageing 1995;24:389-392.
33. Seale C, Addington-Hall J.   Euthanasia: why people want to die earlier.   Soc Sci Med 1994;39:647-654.
34. Owen C, Tennant C, Levi J, et al.   Cancer patients' attitudes to final events in life: wish for death, attitudes to cessation of treatment, suicide and euthanasia.   Psycho-Oncology 1994;3:1-9.
35. Brown JH, Henteleff P, Barakat S, et al.   Is it normal for terminally ill patients to desire death? Am J Psychiatry 1986;143:208-211.
36. Chochinov HM, Wilson K, Enns, M, et al.   Prevalence of depression in the terminally ill: effects of diagnostic criteria and symptom threshold judgments.   Am J Psychiatry 1994;51:537-540.
37. Guze S, Robins E.   Suicide and primary affective disorders.   Br J Psychiatry 1970;47:437-438.
38. Ganzini L, Lee MA, Heintz RT, et al.   The effect of depression treatment on elderly patients' preferences for life-sustaining medical therapy.   Am J Psychiatry 1994;51:1631-1636.
39. Hooper SC, Vaughan KJ, Tennant CC, et al.   Major depression and refusal of life-sustaining medical treatment in the elderly.   MJA 1996;165:416-419.
40. Beck AT, Beck RW.   Screening depressed patients in family practice: a rapid technic.   Postgrad Med 1972;52:81-85.
41. Hooper SC, Vaughan KJ, Tennant CC, et al.   Preferences for voluntary euthanasia during major depression and following improvement in an elderly population.   Australian J Ageing 1997;16:3-7.
42. Keown J. On regulating death. Hastings Cent Rep 1992;22(2):39-43.
43. Chochinov HM, Tataryn D, Dudgeon D, et al.   Will to live in the terminally ill (Abstract). Academy of Psychosomatic (Current Submission).

Depression: a major psychological and emotional problem

Shigeto Yamawaki

Department of Psychiatry and Neuroscience, Hiroshima University School of Medicine
1-2-3, Kasumi, Minami-ku, Hiroshima 734, Japan

SUMMARY OF SESSION

Depression and anxiety are frequently observed in the patients suffering form life threatening disease such as cancer and AIDS. Recently the importance of psycho-social approach to such patients has been recognized in palliative medicine. In this session, psychological and emotional problems, especially depression observed in advanced or terminal cancer patients and HIV-infected patients have been discussed.

Dr. Okamura reported the prevalence of psychiatric disorders in the patients with advanced cancer in Japan. In his investigation using the structured clinical interview(SCID), adjustment disorders with depressive mood and anxiety was observed in 36.4% of recurrent breast cancer patients and in 13.4% of non-small-cell lung cancer patients, and major depression was also observed in 6.8% and 1.0%, respectively. He also reported all 5 patients with terminal cancer who expressed desire for death were diagnosed as major depression, and tricyclic antidepressants improved depressive symptoms of these patients. In the discussion time, the reason why he used tricyclic antidepressants which have an strong anti-cholinergic side effect was questioned. Dr. Okamura answered that a selective serotonin reuptake inhibitors (SSRIs) will be appropriate, but SSRIs are not on market in Japan at present.

Dr. Hollander presented the recent prevalent study on depression in HIV-infected adults. Several initial investigations reported the high incidence of depression in HIV-infected populations, but he commented that these data were exaggerated estimates. He mentioned however there is some evidence that depression may increase the relative risk of CD4 lymphocyte decline, disease progression and mortality. Seventy-five percent of depression in HIV-infected adults may be improved by standard antidepressants like SSRIs, but have a higher rate of adverse reactions due to the presence of underlying nervous system infection. Finally he emphasized that the improving prognosis of HIV disease due to protease inhibitor therapy will have a good effect on emotional problems in this population. One of audience commented the limitation of protease inhibitor therapy and the difficulty of treating with HIV-infected adults in Japan.

Dr. Chochinov presented the issues of under-diagnosis of depression in dying patients. He reported the prevalence of major depression to range from 10 to 17% in a cohort of terminal cancer, and the usefulness of brief screening measures to identify clinical depression amongst the terminally-ill. In his another study, the prevalence of genuine desire for death was 8.5%, which was highly correlated with clinical depression. In the study using a visual analog scale, he found that four main predictors of variance in 'will to live' were depression, anxiety, shortness of breath and sense of well being. In the discussion time, some of audience asked what kind of antidepressants should be recommended to prescribe to depression of terminally-ill. He recommended SSRIs because of low side effect. Finally, Dr. Bruera summarized this session and emphasized the importance of early awareness of depression in advanced cancer and terminally-ill patients, and also of psycho-social support to those populations.

Session IV

Ethics in Palliative Medicine

Chairpersons:
Stephen C. Schimpff and Tetsuro Shimizu

Euthanasia in the Netherlands: A Flat Country On A Slippery Slope?

Geert H. Blijham, M.D.

Professor and Chairman, Department of Medicine, University Hospital Utrecht, P.O. Box 85500, 3508 GA Utrecht, The Netherlands

SUMMARY. In the Netherlands "Medical Decisions Concerning End of Life" (MDEL) play a role in 65% of cancer deaths. Non-treatment decisions occur in 18%, treatment with narcotics that may fasten death in 38% and euthanasia or physician-assisted suicide in 8% of cases. Of Dutch physicians 53% have ever performed euthanasia and only 3% would never perform or refer for euthanasia on moral or religious grounds. Of the 30.000 requests for euthanasia or physician-assisted suicide 10% are eventually granted. In 1993 the Dutch legislation has been reformed. Euthanasia remains a crime and each case will be reviewed by the district attorney. Court discisions, however, have confirmed the view that in cases of euthanasia the physician may be confronted with conflicting obligations and therefore will not be punished. As a consequence, cases fulfilling a number of requirements will not be prosecuted. Comparison between the data from 1990 and 1995 show an increased rate of notification (from 18% tot 41%) without an increase in the percentage of requests that is granted or a shift to less terminal conditions. In the Netherlands euthanasia or physician-assisted suicide are considered ethically justifiable and legally permissible if it is part of an open, honest and careful approach to patients with unbearable suffering, in particular in the case of cancer.

KEY WORDS: Euthanasia, physician-assisted suicide, cancer.

INTRODUCTION

Despite progress in the prevention, early detection and treatment of cancer still around 50% of patients, at least in the Western world, will die from their disease. They at some point have to face the prospect of a lifespan that is much shorter than anticipated, of a gradual decline of functional capabilities and of the possible agony of death. Often from one day to the other the very basis of existence changes and it is understandable that this change is associated with a variety of reactions, from denial through anger and despair to acceptance. Coping with the notion that one's life will end shortly and untimely is extremely variable between individuals and depending on one's unique individual history as well as one's cultural and societal environment. Each discussion of the medical decisions concerning end of life therefore has to start with the recognition of the private aspects of how patients want to lead their remaining life and how they want to prepare for death. More than anywhere else in medicine, the physician caring for dying patients should listen rather than talk, follow rather than lead, understand rather than convince, see the patient rather than the disease. This is not a plea for being passive but rather for the provision of comfort in an active way. It is also a plea for having an open mind in order to prevent that the physician himself, with his own unique history and cultural background, comes between what the patient needs and the doctor can provide. It is this open mind, that characterizes the past and present of the discussion about medical decisions concerning end of life (MDEL), including Euthanasia, in the Netherlands and that should be its main message to the world.

Health Care in the Netherlands

Before presenting and discussing the Euthanasia situation in the Netherlands, it is important to consider the cultural and health care background of this country. It is densely populated with 15 million inhabitants on 30.000 km^2 and a high standard of living. Despite a rich religious history this small nation of international traders has a tradition of openness and a dislike of chauvinism and dogmatism. As far as the health care system is concerned, close to 100% of the population is insured with a coverage of virtually all aspects of care. All individuals belong to the practice of a general practitioner and there are many nursing homes to care for those who cannot be cared for at home. As a consequence of this extensive system of extramural facilities only slightly over one-third of patients die in the hospital and many (40-45%) at home.

Medical Decisions Concerning End of Life (MDEL)

Every day physicians caring for patients with intractable diseases are confronted with dilemma's concerning the prolongation or ending of life. As much as preservation of life is a moral obligation for all doctors, this obligation has its limitations in what the patient considers to be his or her best own interest. MDEL refer to the situation that in the care of patients prolongation or maintenance of life is not the number one priority anymore but gives way to decisions that accept the upcoming death as a fact of life.

In line with van der Maas et al [1] 5 types of MDEL can be observed in daily practice [table 1].

Table 1. Medical Decisions Concerning End of Life: Definitions

Decision not to Treat	The withholding or withdrawal of potentially life-prolonging treatment
Alleviation of Pain and Symtoms with Opoids	The administration of doses large enough that there is a probable life-shortening effect
Euthanasia	The administration of drugs with the explicit intention of ending the patient's life at the patient's explicit request
Physician-Assisted Suicide	The prescription or supply of drugs with the explicit intention of enabling the patient to end his or her own life
Ending of Life without Explicit Request	The administration of drugs with the explicit intention of ending the patient's life without a concurrent, explicit request by the patient

Included in "No-Treatment Decisions" (NTD) is not to give antibiotics to a patient with a terminal cancer and a life expectancy of two weeks, who develops pneumonia. In fact, just because of this, pneumonia is the final cause of deaths in many death statistics. Virtually all physicians will agree on the wisdom of such no-treatment decisions. In the United Kingdom 91% of practitioners and hospital consultants agreed with the withdrawal or withholding of treatment from a terminally ill patient even if knowing that the treatment might prolong the patients life [2].

Some patients suffer from symptoms, that in order to be treated effectively need a potentially dangerous approach. For instance in case of severe pain it may be necessary to push the treatment with morphine to dose levels, that are associated with a real risk of severe respiratory depression and death. "Alleviation of Pain and Symptoms" (APS) is the intended result of such decisions, which are made daily by physicians, preferably in close consultation with their patients. In New England 97% of oncologists, 93% of oncological patients and 92% of the public agreed that in terminal cancer with unremitting pain the morphine dose could be increased to control pain even if premature death is a likely consequence [3].

Physician-assisted termination of life refers to medical acts that have the intention to hasten death and terminate life. This may concern the intravenous injection of high dose barbiturates or muscle relaxants by the doctor (Euthanasia) or the patient taking deathly medicines prescribed by the doctor (Physician-Assisted Suicide, PAS). As long as it concerns a competent patient with an explicit request there is no ethical difference between the two. Some consider physician-assisted suicide to be preferable because of the more active participation by the patient. Given the active role of the doctor in prescribing and often providing the lethal drugs, however, the difference between euthanasia and physician-assisted suicide is mainly a psychological one and has the danger for the latter to become an ethical alibi. Interestingly in a survey in New England oncologists were more likely to support legalisation of physician-assisted suicide (supported by 43% of oncologists) than of euthanasia (35%). For patients and the public the opposite was true (59%-57% versus 70%-66%) [3].

The most controversial, finally, are physician-assisted life terminating acts related to incompetent patients, such as baby's, those with dementia or terminal cancer patients slipping into a state of somnolence, confusion or even coma. The Dutch definition of euthanasia excludes those patients ("explicit request by a competent patient").

The Incidence of Euthanasia and other MDEL in the Netherlands

In 1990 Dutch researchers started an investigation into the incidence and characteristics of MDEL in the Netherlands [1]. In 1995 this investigation was repeated with the intent to monitor a possible change in the incidence and reporting of euthanasia and PAS after the introduction of new legislation [4]. In both investigations two sources of data were explored. A random sample of around 400 practising physicians from a variety of disciplines were interviewed with a 120 page questionnaire; the response rate was 89%. At the same time of stratified sample of over 6000 death certificates were examined; physicians responsible for these certificates received an anonymous 24-items questionnaire of which 77% were returned. Results from the interview and death certificate approach were almost overlapping; in the following discussion these data will be taken together.

Table 2. Medical Decisions Concerning End of Life in the Netherlands

	1990	1995	1995 (cancer)
Decision not to treat	18%	20%	18%
Alleviation of pain	19%	19%	38%
Physician-assisted suicide	0,2%	0,2%	0,6%
Euthanasia	1,7%	2,4%	7%
Ending Life without explicit request	0,8%	0,7%	1%
All	39%	43%	65%

Table 2 gives the incidence of the 5 types of MDEL as percentages of all deaths in 1990 and 1995 and for deaths due to cancer in 1995. A number of conclusions can be drawn. MDEL play a role in around 40% of all deaths and 65% of cancer deaths. NTD and APS each occurs in around 19% of deaths and this has not changed between 1990 and 1995. Euthanasia and PAS are rare events and have increased slightly between 1990 and 1995 from 1.9% to 2.6%. Ending of life without explicit request is even more rare with 1% or around 1000 cases per year. In cancer patients MDEL, in particular the use of opioids that may have hastened death and euthanasia, occur more frequently than in patients dying from other causes.

Attitudes of patients and doctors towards Euthanasia and PAS

The design of the study by van der Maas et al made it possible to estimate the actual frequency of euthanasia in relation to how often patients bring up the possibility and a request is made [table 3]. Per year around 35.000 Dutch patients seeks assurance from their doctors that they will assist them in case suffering becomes unbearable. Of these, 10,000 eventually have an explicit request for euthanasia and 3700 are agreed to. In the other cases alternatives are found that make life bearable again and in other instances the patient dies before any action has to be taken.

Table 3. Euthanasia and PAS in the Netherlands: Patient Requests

	1990	1995
number of patients	128,786	135,546
number of requests for Euthanasia or PAS later in the disease	25,100	34,500
number of explicit requests for Euthanasia or PAS	8900	9700
number of deaths resulting from Euthanasia or PAS	2833	3660

Apparently many patients bring up euthanasia or other MDEL; what is the attitude of Dutch doctors towards these requests [table 4]. Of the 400 physicians interviewed around 50% had ever performed and around one-third were willing to perform euthanasia under certain circumstances. Apparently the large majority of physicians in the Netherlands see euthanasia as an accepted element of medical practice under certain circumstances. In fact, only 3-4% of physicians would never perform euthanasia or refer for it. There were no major differences between general practitioners, medical specialists and nursing home doctors in this respect.

Table 4. Euthanasia in the Netherlands: Doctor's Attitudes

Euthanasia	1990 (%)	1995 (%)
ever performed	54	53
willing to perform	34	29
refusal but referral	8	9
total refusal	4	3

In contrasf to what is sometimes believed, the data show that euthanasia is a rare event in the Netherlands and is finally done in around 10% of those who have brought it up and in around 7% of all patients dying from cancer. The attitude towards euthanasia, however, is an open one with more than 50% of the physicians practising medicine having ever performed it and with less than 5% who will never do it nor refer patients for this purpose to another physician. These figures have certainly influenced the decisions of the goverment regarding euthanasia, that recently have passed both houses of parliament and will be discussed briefly.

The Dutch Legislation on Euthanasia

In the past as well as today in the Netherlands euthanasia according to the definition given is a crime and the physician performing euthanasia is formally open to criminal prosecution with a maximal punishment of 12 years in prison. In recent years, however, a number of court decisions have confirmed the view, that in cases of euthanasia the physician may be confronted with conflicting obligations. His professional obligations may lead him to act in accordance with the explicit wish of his patient; the patient expressing this wish trusts that the physician will perform euthanasia in order to allow the patient whose suffering is unbearable and cannot be relieved, to die in dignity. However, in doing so the physician will act against the formal provisions of the law, that he has to follow as a civilian. In that situation of conflicting obligations the courts have ruled, that the physician will be judged guilty without punishment provided he performs euthanasia according to certain rules.

Based upon this jurisprudence the Royal Dutch Medical Association developed a set of requirements, that a physician has to meet in performing euthanasia. These 5 requirements, which all should be met, are given in table 5.

Table 5. Requirements for Physician-Assisted Death in The Netherlands

---

- the patient must consider his or her suffering unbearable and hopeless

- there is a well considered and persistent wish to die

- the request must be voluntary

- the physician must consult at least one other physician

Between 1984 and 1990, these requirements were confirmed in court decisions. However, physicians could still be and sometimes were prosecuted. Therefore many cases of euthanasia were not reported and the death was classified as natural. This was the main reason to start the study of 1990 with the purpose to obtain reliable estimates of the occurrence of euthanasia and its characteristics.

Reassured by the findings of the investigation and based upon the broad consensus within the population and the professionals, new legislation passed both houses of parliament in 1993. This legislation may be considered somewhat bizar in the sense that it only concerns procedures and does not in any way decriminalize or legalize euthanasia. Termination of life of a severely suffering patient on his or her request by a doctor remains a crime and the Penal Code has not been changed. The Bill is no more than an Amendment to the Burial Act with the effect, that a special notification procedure will be laid down in the regulations under this Act and will thereby acquire formal legal status. It now becomes possible to formally report euthanasia including the circumstances under which it took place. However, under which circumstances the physician will not be prosecuted remains based upon jurisprudence. This solution offers for the district attorney the possibility to start investigations and prosecution if he deems this appropriate and on the other hand makes it possible for the physician to safely report euthanasia if it is conducted according to good medical practice as based upon previous court decisions. The current notification procedure is depicted in table 6. With this new legislation the percentage of cases of physician-assisted death reported to the authorities increased from 18% in 1990 to 41% in 1995 [5]. In these years 13 of 6324 reported cases (0.2%) were prosecuted; 6 physicians were sentenced.

Table 6: Notification Procedure for Physician-Assisted Death

• no certificate of natural death

• physician informs the coroner of a physician-assisted death

• physician fills in an offical checklist with questions about:
- medical history
- the request of the patient
- the drugs used to cause death
- report of consulted physician

• coroner collects the data and informs the public prosecutor

• prosecutor examines the data and:
- permits burial or cremation
- presents a judgement to the prosecutor general

• the data are examined in the Assembly of Prosecutors General which decides whether or not to prosecute

• final decision about prosecution by the Minister of Justice.

1990 agreed between Medical Association and Minister, legal since 1994 as an Amendment to the Burial Act

A Flat Country on a Slippery Slope?

In the Netherlands, around 0,7% of all deaths occur as a result of a life-terminating act without an actual explicit request [4]. This figure, obtained in a country with free access for every one to high level oncological and palliative care, has attracted much attention. It has been made less clear, that many of these patients (52%) prior to their state of incompetence had expressed strong opinions about euthanasia, that older patients were under- rather than overrepresented and that virtually all (91%) were in such terminal phase of their disease that the life expectancy was considered to be less than one week. Also, doctors in the Netherlands felt more reluctant regarding life-terminating acts without explicit request. Twenty-three percent had ever done it and another 32% would do it under certain circumstances, figures that are considerably lower than for euthanasia.

Concern about the "1000 people killed without consent each year in the Netherlands" also plays a role in the slippery slope argument. It says that by allowing physician-assisted suicide and euthanasia, underprivileged, impaired or undertreated patients may run the risk to be killed. It also may constitute an "easy way out" for doctors who do not have the time, skills or inclination to care for dying patients. A comparison between the figures from 1990 and 1995 may help to address the Slippery Slope argument. They show that actually apart from the increased percentage of notification little has changed [table 7]. In particular the percentage of requests granted and the percentage of patients in a terminal condition has not changed. It can be argued that in fact the Dutch openness about MDEL is one of the best safeguards against abuse and the development of a slippery slope.

Table 7. Slippery Slope for Physician-Assisted Death in the Netherlands?

	1990	1995
• percentage of request that is granted, is stable	27%	32%
• percentage of deaths due to ending of life without explicit request, is decreasing	0,8%	0,7%
• cancer remains the main diagnosis	68%	61%
• no shift to less terminal conditions (shorterning of life > 1 wk)	43%	41%
• more consultation and notification	18%	41%

Conclusion

In the Netherlands, 30,000 patients per year discuss euthanasia and physician-assisted suicide with their doctors, 10000 of these eventually have an explicit request and 3000 are granted [4]. This illustrates that euthanasia is not an isolated request at the end of a fatal disease, but part of the journey of doctor and patient towards the inevitable end of life. In my department, around 5 cancer patients per year will die as a result of a granted euthanasia request. This is never an "easy way out" but the final outcome of an always careful, sometimes agonizing but often gratifying process involving patients, families, doctors and nurses. Oncologists should know about the ethical, legal and practical aspects of life-terminating acts as part of their experience in the care for dying patients with cancer. They should also be experts in palliative care, a role they have indeed taken on given the attention for supportive and palliative care in the major oncological journals and conferences [6]. With this dual expertise they can testify to the important notion that euthanasia does not exclude good palliative care nor should good palliative care exclude euthanasia. This same dual expertise could also provide the best safeguard against the development of a slippery slope in how we, as physicians caring for terminal cancer patients, deal with the inevitable dilemma's of life and death.

REFERENCES

1. van der Maas PJ, van Delden JJM, Pijnenborg L et al (1991) Euthanasia and other medical decisions concerning the end of life. Lancet 338:669-74.
2. Ward BJ, Tate PA (1994) Attitudes among NHS doctors to requests for euthanasia. BMJ 308:1332-4.
3. Emanuel EJ, Fairclough DL, Daniels ER et al (1996) Euthanasia and physician-assisted suicide: Attitudes and experiences of oncology patients, oncologists, and the public. Lancet 347:1805-10.
4. van der Maas PJ, van der Wal G, Haverkate I et al (1996) Euthanasia, Physician-Assisted Suicide, and other Medical Practice involving the End of Life in the Netherlands, 1990-1995. NEJM 335:1699-1705.
5. van der Wal G, van der Maas PJ, Bosma JM et al (1996) Evaluation of the notification procedure for physician-assisted death in the Netherlands. NEJM 335:1706-1711.
6. Blijham GH (1996) Euthanasia, physician-assisted suicide and palliative care. Ann Oncol 7:879-882.

Evaluation of Do-Not-Resuscitate Policy in Japan

Asato Fukaura

First Department of Internal Medicine, Showa University School of Medicine, 1-5-8 Hatanodai, Shinagawa-ku, Tokyo 142 JAPAN

SUMMARY. The use of cardiopulmonary resuscitation (CPR) must be carefully considered, especially for terminally ill and elderly patients. The use of DNR orders is relatively new to Japan and there has been little discussion of DNR policy. In 1994, we introduced standardized DNR order forms and guidelines at our university hospital. This study found that CPR was performed much less often after the introduction of the DNR order forms than before in patients who died of lung cancer. This finding might reflect both educational efforts and greater awareness of DNR due to the introduction and use of DNR orders and guidelines. Although few competent patients participated in DNR decisions, surrogates or proxies were consulted in all cases. Because advance directives for medical care have not yet been advocated in Japan, we surveyed inpatients and found that they preferred to participate in decisions about life-sustaining treatment if they could discuss their decision with physicians. Therefore, we introduced an original advance directive called the Personal Medical Directive which can serve as a tool for discussion. Medical opinions on the appropriateness of CPR for certain patients should now be openly discussed. Further efforts to improve both patient participation in decision-making and DNR practice are recommended. We continue to strive for concrete measures, such as the introduction of DNR order forms and the Personal Medical Directive, to improve terminal care and to give all patients an equal opportunity to benefit from medical care.

KEY WORDS: do-not-resuscitate order, cardiopulmonary resuscitation, advance directive, proxy, life-sustaining treatment

INTRODUCTION

The use of cardiopulmonary resuscitation (CPR) must be carefully considered, especially for terminally ill and elderly patients [1-8] for whom dying should not be unnecessarily prolonged. Accordingly, there has been considerable discussion about do-not-resuscitate (DNR) orders in North America [9-15], Europe [16-20], and other areas [21-23]. However, because medical practice and ethics in Japan differ from those elsewhere, there has been comparatively little discussion and few studies of DNR policy in Japan [24,25]. However, physicians, even if Japanese, are often forced to consider how CPR and DNR orders are performed. Although physicians usually practice medicine in accordance with their own ethical standards, how DNR orders are used is unknown. Therefore, when and why orders are written, who had been consulted about the order, and how the orders were carried out should be investigated to find out possible problems with DNR orders and terminal care in Japan.

In this paper, we present results of our studies of the practice of DNR after introduction of a DNR policy at our teaching hospital in Japan and of problems with the decision-making process for life-sustaining treatment. We also introduce a new advance directive to address these problems.

AWARENESS OF DNR ORDERS AMONG JAPANESE PHYSICIANS

The use of DNR orders is relatively new to Japan and few studies of DNR orders have been performed. We surveyed awareness of the DNR principle among Japanese physicians (n=352) with a nationwide questionnaire [26].

Most physicians answering the questionnaire felt that resuscitation of patients with terminal lung cancer is inappropriate (96%) and most had consulted others concerning DNR orders (96%). Ceremonial resuscitation was often performed until all family members had arrived at the bedside (46%), even though 40% of respondents felt that resuscitation should ideally be performed according to the patient's wishes. Despite the high awareness of the principle of DNR, futile CPR is often performed at the time of death in terminal lung cancer patients.

We found that although physicians feel resuscitation of patients with terminal lung cancer is inappropriate, aggressive resuscitation is occasionally performed. Furthermore, despite most physicians' being aware of and having written DNR orders, ceremonial resuscitation is still performed.

INTRODUCTION OF DNR POLICY

In a retrospective study of 75 deaths from lung cancer at our teaching hospital from 1990 through 1992, ceremonial and futile resuscitations were also performed (Arai T: personal communication). We suspect that reasons futile resuscitation is performed so often include the lack of a uniform DNR policy and poor communication of DNR orders among medical staff. However, we could still not determine how DNR orders are carried out.

A DNR policy at an institution reduces the incidence of resuscitative efforts in terminally ill patients and increases the prevalence of patients who receive DNR orders before death [27,28]. Because our hospital and other institutions in Japan had no official DNR policy, we held discussions and developed original guidelines for DNR orders in 1994 (Table 1) [43]. A DNR order form was also created (Fig. 1). We believe that this easily used standard form improves documentation of DNR orders and reduces misunderstandings that often occur when physicians fail to clearly and fully communicate treatment plans to the other members of the treatment staff [29-31].

Table 1. Summary of the basic principles of the DNR guidelines

---

1. Active euthanasia should not be allowed under any circumstances.

2. The DNR order does not mean withdrawing personal attention from the patient or limiting attention to the relief of suffering.

3. The wishes of an informed patient who can make decisions should be the primary consideration in all DNR decisions.

4. Unless a DNR order indicates otherwise, it is presumed that life-sustaining interventions, including CPR, will be provided.

5. Clear discussions among health professionals, patients, and patients' surrogates should be held to make DNR decisions.

6. It is the physician's responsibility to provide the patient or surrogate with adequate information about therapeutic and diagnostic options, so that the patient or surrogate can make an informed decision.

7. When a decision is made to proceed with a DNR order, the order should be entered on the DNR order sheet by the physician responsible for the patient's care.

8. DNR orders should be reviewed as needed. If the order is to be renewed or changed in any way, a new order sheet must be completed immediately.

9. The ultimate responsibility for implementation of this policy rests with the patient's private physician.

10. The DNR order form is not a legal document.

DNR order sheet   vol.

DO NOT RESUSCITATE

In the event of a cardiopulmonary arrest, no resuscitative measures will be initiated.

_____ **no intubation**

_____ **no mechanical ventilation**

_____ **no chest compression**

_____ **no tracheotomy**

_____ **no Ambu Cardiopump**

_____ **no defibrillation**

_____ **other**

DATE:	TIME:	Physician's Signature:

1 Diagnosis: _____

2 **The documented reasons for the DNR order (check all that apply):**

_____ condition irreversible, deaths imminent (within 2 weeks)

_____ condition irreversible, limited life expectancy (within 6 months)

_____ unacceptable quality of life

_____ requested by patient

_____ requested by family

_____ other

3 Patient competency: competent

_____ incompetent

_____ variable

4 Discussion of DNR order has occurred with (check all that apply):

_____ patient

_____ family (specify _____)

_____ nursing stuff

_____ private physician

_____ other
DISCONTINUED ABOVE ORDERS IMMEDIATELY Reasons to discontinue the orders:
DATE:　　　TIME:　　　Physician's Signature:

Fig. 1.　Structured DNR order sheet

This prospective study evaluated the use of a standardized DNR order form and its effect on CPR in three inpatient units (with a total of 90 beds) of the First Department of Internal Medicine, Showa University Hospital, from January 1 through December 31, 1994. The selected medical units did not include intensive care units and hospices. A DNR order could be written with a standardized form (Fig. 1) for any inpatient of the three units aged 16 years or older who met the criteria of our DNR policy. A DNR order could proscribe any or all CPR procedures, including intubation, mechanical ventilation, chest compression, tracheotomy, Ambu cardiopump, and defibrillation. The following information was collected from medical records, DNR order forms, and physicians of each patient who died: (1) age; (2) sex; (3) principal diagnosis; (4) CPR procedures permitted at the time of an arrest; (5) reasons for the DNR order; (6) involvement of patients, surrogates (family members), or hospital staff in the DNR decision; (7) mental status of the patient; (8) performance of CPR at death; and (9) presence of assigned physician and family at death.

EVALUATION OF USING DNR POLICY

During the study period 443 patients were admitted. Of the 56 patients (13%) who had received DNR orders, 48 died and 8 were alive at the end of study period and were discharged to home or another facility. Nineteen patients died without receiving DNR orders. Therefore, 48 (71.6%) of the 67 patients who died had received DNR orders. The percentage of patients who had received DNR orders before death is similar to those reported in other countries (61% to 68%) [9,12,15,20,21].

Patients who received DNR orders were generally older men who had malignancies (75%), especially lung cancer (57%), and were incompetent (55%). Uhlman et al showed age to be an independent predictor of DNR orders [32]. The current study showed that although 83% (5 of 6) of patients who were aged 80 years or older had received DNR orders before death, 61% of patients aged less than 60 years (11 of 18) also died with DNR orders. Although accurately predicting time of death is difficult, physicians should be encouraged to apply DNR orders uniformly in patients with different diseases but with similar prognoses [33]. However, in our study, patients who died with DNR orders were significantly more likely to have cancer (77%) than were patients who died without DNR orders (32%). This difference may also explain why older patients were more likely to have DNR orders since older patients were also more likely to have cancer.

In most cases, DNR orders were written either more than 1 month (34%) or within 3 days (32%) before the patient died. Furthermore, 82% of patients received only a single DNR order. At first, this finding might appear to indicate good decision-making processes. However, we believe it suggests that once a DNR order was written, it was rarely reconsidered. Studies in other countries have also found that the purpose and timing of DNR decisions were rarely reevaluated [10,34]. Although the DNR guidelines call for the order to be reconsidered if the patient's condition changes, this was infrequently done.   One possible reason for this lack of reevaluation is that the use of DNR orders is not yet common in Japan and problems with their use might be expected.

In our study, imminent death (within 2 weeks) and limited life expectancy (less than 6 months) were the stated reasons for the DNR order in 38% and 34% of cases, respectively.   Unacceptable quality of life was the stated reason in only 18% of cases.   Since the present study did not investigate how physicians or family discussed the DNR decision, we do not know to what extent patients' quality of life was actually considered.   The patient's family requested the DNR order in 45% of cases, compared with only 11% of cases in which the patient requested the order.   Although six patients had expressed a wish to discuss DNR orders, only three (5%) actually participated in the DNR decision.   Instead, surrogates participated in all cases.   In other countries the rates of participation in the DNR decisions were: competent patients, 14% to 41%; surrogates, 33% to 91%; and other medical staff, 6% to 70% [9,12-15,20].

What factors may contribute to the low rate of patient participation in our study?   One reason may be that in Japan, most physicians are hesitant to discuss DNR orders with patients, perhaps because they believe that they already know their patients' preferences regarding resuscitation or because they are concerned that such discussions might create undue patient anxiety.   However, physicians cannot learn their patients' attitudes about terminal care without frank discussions with the patients themselves [14].   In this study, only 35% of patients who died of cancer were told their diagnoses. However, a public-opinion poll and our previous study of medical ethics revealed that more than 60% of both the Japanese public and outpatients want to be told of a diagnosis of cancer and want to die a natural death without aggressive life-sustaining treatments [5,36].   In addition, 46% of Japanese approve of living wills, and 73% support advance directives for the designation of surrogate decision-makers [35].   Advance directives for medical care and the designation of surrogate decision-makers to guide medical care after a patient has become incompetent have not yet been advocated in Japan. Moreover, informing a patient of a diagnosis of cancer is not common in Japan, and other medical ethical issues surrounding DNR orders, such as informed consent and advance directive, are still controversial [25,37-42].

Our study found that resuscitative efforts differed significantly when the family and physician were present and when they were absent (Table 2).   When both family members and private physicians were absent, resuscitative efforts were both more aggressive and more frequently performed than when either family members or private physicians were present.   We speculate that this finding may indicate that CPR is often performed when family members are absent in an attempt to keep the patient alive until family members arrive.   When the family members were present, CPR was less aggressive or not performed at all, and the patient was allowed to die without intervention.

Table 2.   Summary of comparison of the CPR procedures permitted on the DNR order sheet with those actually performed in the 48 patients with DNR orders who died.

Situation	No CPR permitted	CPR procedures permitted		
		Intubation	chest compression	Ambu cardiopump
Family, physician, or both absent (n=15)				
Permitted on sheet	4 (27)	2 (13)	5 (33)	8 (53)
Actually performed	5 (33)	4 (27)	4 (27)	9 (60)
P value		0.01		

Family and physician

both present (n=33)				
Permitted on sheet	13 (39)	3 (9)	12 (36)	19 (58)
Actually performed	21 (64)	2 (6)	8 (24)	10 (30)
P value	0.03			<0.001
All cases (n=48)				
Permitted on sheet	17 (35)	5 (11)	17 (35)	27 (56)
Actually performed	26 (54)	6 (13)	12 (25)	19 (40)
P value	0.007			0.02

Numbers followed by a number in parentheses are numbers of patients and percentages of the group. Only P values less than 0.05 are shown.
Percentages may not add to a hundred percent because of rounding.

Physicians' attitudes regarding discussions of DNR orders with patients are no doubt more complex and resistant to change than our results suggest. We believe that physicians should educate all chronically ill and seriously ill patients about their options regarding life-sustaining treatment and provide a supportive environment in which these patients may feel comfortable expressing their preferences [10]. Further study of DNR orders and other medical ethical issues in Japan is needed.

However, this study found that CPR was performed much less often after the introduction of the DNR order form (41% of cases) than before (91%, Arai T; personal communication) in patients who died of lung cancer (Table 3). This finding might reflect both educational efforts and greater awareness of DNR after introduction and use of the DNR order form and DNR guidelines. Our DNR order form and DNR policy could be adapted for use by other institutions. Hospital and community education projects that involve the Japanese public in discussions of DNR would increase patient participation in DNR decisions. An official DNR policy would decrease misunderstanding between physicians and patients. Discussions about the medical decisions concerning the end of life should no longer be secret.

Table 3. Comparison of the CPR procedures to lung cancer patients deaths before and after using the DNR order sheet

Situation	No CPR	CPR procedures		
		Intubation	Chest compression	Ambu cardiopump
Before using DNR order sheet (n=75)	9	43	87	85
After using DNR order sheet (n=25)	59	4	19	37
P value	<.0001	<.0001	<.0001	<.0001

All figures indicate percentages of patients.

INPATIENTS' PREFERENCES OF DECISION-MAKING PROCESS

Some medical inpatients are in realistic state to discuss medical ethical problems, such as treatment choices, life-sustaining treatments, DNR orders, and proxy decision making. Our previous studies revealed that in Japan, orders, such as DNR orders, to limit or withdraw life-sustaining treatments are widely but secretly used and that decisions about DNR orders are usually made by proxies or surrogates rather than by patients [26,43]. These findings raise several questions. Do inpatients want to participate in the decision-making process? Whose opinion do they want to follow regarding treatment? Whom should they select as proxies? What do patients think about life-sustaining treatments? Are patients willing to discuss life-sustaining treatments?

To determine medical inpatients' preferences in making decisions about treatment choices, we performed an in-person survey using two types of multiple-choice questionnaire [49]. Each questionnaire consisted of 12 questions designed to determine inpatients' personal profile: 1) age, 2) sex, 3) working or retired, 4) marital status, 5) highest level of education, 6) religion, 7) worry about medical fees, and 8) previous admission to this hospital. Eligible participants were asked the following questions. 1) Whose opinion do you want to follow in making decisions about treatments choices? 2) Whom do you want to be with you when your physical condition and examination results are explained so that they can serve as proxy? 3) How do you think and decide about taking life-sustaining treatments?

We used two kinds of multiple-choice questionnaires: phase 1 (P-1) and phase 2 (P-2). The two questionnaires differed in only one sentence, "Wish to decide by myself" (P-1) to "Wish to decide by myself after discussion with my physician" (P-2), which were designed to find out whether patients wish to discuss medical problems with their physicians. This survey was conducted every 4 months from January 4 through April 30, 1995, for P-l, and from 14 May 1 through August 31, 1995, for P-2. This study involved inpatients on the units of the First Department of Internal Medicine at Showa University Hospital, which are the same units using the DNR order form. During each study period all new inpatients were surveyed within 2 weeks after admission. To be considered eligible, inpatients had to be able to speak and to hear and to be allowed by their physicians to participate. A questionnaire was conducted by the authors and all patients consented to participate.

Of the 283 new inpatients (P-1, 143; P-2, 140), 166 (58.7%) (P-1, 96; P-2, 70) completed a questionnaire during the study period. The P-1 and P-2 patients had similar socioeconomic characteristics, except that the P-2 patients were slightly more highly educated and had more often been hospitalized (Table 4). In P-1, 58 patients (60%) answered that they would follow their physicians' opinion in making decisions regarding treatment choices. In P-2, 40 patients (57%) answered that they would wish to decide by themselves after discussions with their physicians (Table 5). In P-1, 47 patients (49%) preferred to die naturally, but in P-2, 40 patients (57%) preferred to discuss life-sustaining treatments with their physicians.

Table 4. Socioeconomic characteristics of the patients

Characteristics		Phase 1 (%)	Phase 2 (%)	p value
No of patients		96	70	
Sex	Male	51 (53)	37 (53)	
	Female	45 (47)	33 (47)	
Age, y	<40	11 (11)	15 (21)	
	41-59	30 (31)	24 (34)	
	51-79	48 (50)	28 (40)	
	80<	7 (7)	3 (4)	
	mean ± SD	54.6 ± 19.1	58.0 ± 16.1	
	range	17-93	23-87	
Working		47(49)	38 (54)	
Retired		49 (51)	32 (46)	
Marital status				
	Married	79 (82)	52 (74)	

	Unmarried	17 (18)	18 (26)	
Highest education				
	Junior High	23 (24)	9 (13)	0.04
	Senior High	33 (34)	30 (43)	
	College	32 (33)	25 (36)	
	Others	8 (8)	6 (9)	
Religion				
	Atheist	60 (63)	44 (63)	
	Buddhist	28 (32)	24 (34)	
	Others	8 (5)	2 (3)	
Do you worry about the payment?				
	Yes	28 (29)	23 (33)	
	No	68 (71)	47 (67)	
Admission	First time	45 (47)	46 (66)	0.007
	Twice or more	51 (53)	24 (34)	
Diagnosis	Respiratory disease	34 (35)	24 (34)	
	Lung cancer	19 (20)	8 (11)	
	Other cancer	5 (5)	1 (1)	
	Others	38 (40)	37 (53)	

Numbers followed by a number in parentheses are numbers of patients and percentages of the group.
Only P values less than 0.05 are shown.
Percentages may not add to a hundred percent because of rounding.

Table 5.   Results of inpatients' preferences of decision-making process about treatment choices

Variable	Phase-1 (%) (n=96)	Phase-2 (%) (n=70)	p value
1. Whose opinion do you want to follow in decision-making of your treatments choices?			
Physician	58 (60)	27 (39)	0.002
Family	5 (5)	1 (1)	
Wish to decide by myself	27 (28)	-	
Wish to decide by myself after discussion with physician	-	40 (57)	
Unsure	4 (4)	1 (1)	
Others	2 (2)	1 (1)	
2. Who do you want to be explained of your physical conditions and results of any medical examinations with?			
Family	67 (70)	49 (70)	
Yourself	28 (29)	20 (29)	
others	1 (1)	1 (1)	
3. How do you think and want to decide about taking life-sustaining treatments?			
As much as possible	4 (4)	1 (1)	
Death with dignity	47 (49)	21 (30)	0.005
Wish to decide by myself	30 (31)	-	
Wish to decide by myself after discussion with physician	-	40 (57)	

Unsure	6 (6)	7 (10)
Others	9 (9)	1 (1)

Numbers followed by a number in parentheses are numbers of patients and percentages of the group.
Only P values less than 0.05 are shown.
Percentages may not add to a hundred percent because of rounding.

Results of this study suggest that patients may not wish their treatment to be decided by only their family or physician but prefer to participate and discuss even life-sustaining treatments with their physician. We have to devise a strategy cautiously because this study was limited to the early stage of admission. Patients must not be excluded from the decision-making process in a medical practice based on informed consent [46]. Although the tendency of authoritarian physicians to not tell patients their diagnoses is based on cultural and religious traditions, physicians should begin to recognize patients' preferences for participating in decision making [47].

OFFERING ADVANCE DIRECTIVES

Even in Japan, we believe that patients should not be excluded from decision making in a patient-centered medical practice based on informed consent. We surveyed inpatients' preferences in the decision-making process and found that they preferred to participate in decisions about life-sustaining treatment if they could discuss the decision with their physicians. Communication among physicians, patients, and family, although essential for a good patient-physician relationship, is often poor [14]. If patients prefer to participate in decision-making, we believe that advance directives might be adapted for them to do so.

Japanese rarely present advance directives. Unless patients state their preferences in advance, physician-selected proxies might decide against actions that patients themselves would choose. A simple type of personal advance directive for use in hospitals would greatly improve the patient-physician relationship [48,51]. Therefore, we introduced an original advance directive called the Personal Medical Directive (PMD) which provides patients the opportunity to communicate to physicians their preferences concerning medical treatment [50] (Fig. 2). The PMD also allows patients and their families to consider and discuss their attitudes about end-of-life medical care.

PERSONAL MEDICAL DIRECTIVE			

1. If you have cancer, do you want to know?   YES   NO   UNSURE
2. If you become terminally ill, do you want to know how much longer you will live?
                                       YES   NO   UNSURE
3. If you are unable to make decisions for yourself, is there any proxies to express your opinion?
                                       YES   NO   UNSURE

4. If you suffer an illness with one of the four possibilities of recovery, which specific treatments are you willing to receive?

Possibilities of Recovery

Treatment	less than 5%			25%			50%			more than 75%		
Antibiotics	yes	no	unsure	yes	no	unsure	yes	no	unsure	yes	no	unsure
Anti-												

neoplastics	yes	no	unsure	yes	no	unsure	yes	no	unsure	yes	no	unsure
Major-operation	yes	no	unsure	yes	no	unsure	yes	no	unsure	yes	no	unsure
Morphine	yes	no	unsure	yes	no	unsure	yes	no	unsure	yes	no	unsure
Mechanical-ventilation	yes	no	unsure	yes	no	unsure	yes	no	unsure	yes	no	unsure

Fig. 2. Structured personal medical directive

Outpatients under the care of the First Department of Internal Medicine at Showa University Hospital were surveyed from February through April 1996 after giving their consent. The attending physician gave patients the PMD to state their preferences regarding truth-telling and proxies and a questionnaire that asked whether advance directives, such as the PMD, were desirable. The patients were also asked about their specific preferences with respect to receiving antibiotics, antineoplastic agents, major surgery, morphine, and mechanical ventilation under each of four possibilities of recovery: less than 5%, 25%, 50%, and more than 75%. The chance of recovery was indicated by a percentage, because we believe that this was the only way to reduce discrepancies and misunderstanding among physicians, patients, and families about the severity of the patients' illness. Using percentages would avoid use of such words as "serious," "critical," and "terminal," which may be interpreted in various ways. The preferences given in the PMD were only for the purpose of our investigation and were not intended to guide treatment.

A total of 231 patients filled out the PMD and the questionnaires (response rate, 97%), and 141 patients (61%) did so completely. Fifty-nine percent of respondents were men and 41% were women. Thirteen percent of outpatients were visiting our hospital for the first time and 85% had visited two or more times.

Table 6. Results of preferences in the Personal Medical Directive.*

1. If you have cancer, do you want to know?

	YES	NO	UNSURE
	70	15	15

2. If you become terminally ill, do you want to know how much longer you will live?

	YES	NO	UNSURE
	68	18	12

3. If you are unable to make decisions for yourself, is there any proxies to express your opinion?

	YES	NO	UNSURE
	80	7	13

4. If you suffer an illness with one of the four possibilities of recovery, which specific treatments are you willing to receive?

Possibilities of Recovery

Treatment	less than 5%			25%			50%			more than 75%		
	yes	no	unsure	yes	no	unsure	yes	no	unsure	yes	no	unsure
Antibiotics	32	48	20	50	21	29	74	9	17	86	5	9
Anti-neoplastics	9	69	22	15	54	31	47	26	27	58	23	19
Major-operation	12	69	19	21	49	30	61	19	20	76	14	10
Morphine	69	13	18	65	11	24	67	11	22	66	15	19
Mechanical-ventilation	10	76	14	13	63	24	41	34	25	52	26	22

All figures indicate percentages of patients.
Percentages may not add to a hundred percent because of rounding.
*Only the patients who could completely answered PMD (141 patients) were calculated.

The results showed that treatments fell into three categories related to prognosis: 1) treatments, such as morphine, desired in any situation; 2) treatments, such as antineoplastic agents, major surgery, and mechanical ventilation, desired if the chance of recovery was more than 50%; and 3) treatments, such as antibiotics, whose desirability increased with the possibility of recovery (Table 6). These findings suggest that the PMD is practical and that its consistency should now be evaluated.

Sixty-one percent of patients filled out the PMD completely. However, the greatest barrier to advance directives is a lack of physician initiative, because patients' knowledge of and experience with such directives are limited [44,45]. Patients with higher levels of education are more likely to write advance directives [45]. In this study, the older the patients were, the less likely they were to complete the PMD (data not shown). This finding suggests that the PMD is not practical for all patients and should be used carefully, especially with elderly patients. Therefore, physician should not force patients to complete a PMD. Although the physician1s initiative is essential, the patient's autonomy in decision making must be respected.

No specific study of advance directives has been performed in Japan. However, most outpatients (77%) had a favorable opinion of the PMD. Some studies have found that although the execution of advance directives alone will not change advance care planning, advance directives have little adverse effect upon health status [52-55]. Further study of advanced directives, such as the PMD, is needed in Japan.

CONCLUSION

Our previous study revealed a high level of awareness of DNR orders among Japanese physicians and found that the introduction of a DNR policy and guidelines in our Japanese teaching hospital reduced the frequency of CPR in lung cancer patients [26,43]. The extent of resuscitative efforts differed substantially depending on whether family members and the physician were present. However, few patients participated in the decision about their own DNR orders. Because our study was performed in only one teaching hospital, further studies are needed to increase awareness of "futile" resuscitation among physicians and patients.

Our study also found that most patients prefer to participate in and discuss decisions, including those concerning life-sustaining treatments, with their physicians [49]. However, patients should not be excluded from decision making in a patient-centered medical practice based on informed consent. Although the tendency of authoritarian physicians to not tell patients their diagnoses is based on cultural and religious traditions, physicians should begin to recognize patients' preferences for participating in decision making [36,46,47]. We have to devise a strategy cautiously, such as the PMD, because this study was limited to the early stage of admission.

We must continue to strive for concrete measures, such as the introduction of DNR order forms and the PMD, to establish improved terminal care and to give all patients the equal opportunity to benefit from medical care. Medical opinions on the appropriateness and futility of CPR for certain patients are still controversial but should now be openly discussed, especially in Japan.

ACKNOWLEDGMENTS

We are indebted to our colleagues of the First Department of Internal Medicine, Showa University School of Medicine, especially Drs. Hiroki Tazawa, Tadashi Arai, Ikuyo Sato, Takashi Hirose, Toshio Mochizuki, Sachiko Hashimoto, Toru Ohmori, Tsukasa Ohnishi, Keita Kasahara, Hisashi Noguchi, Hiroaki Nakajima, and Mitsuru Adachi for their advice and for allowing us to study their patients, and to the administrative staff of the First Internal Medicine Unit at Showa University Hospital.

REFERENCES

1. Tomlinson T, Brody H (1988) Ethics and communication in do-not-resuscitate orders.   N Engl J Med 318:43-46
2. American Heart Association Committee on Cardiopulmonary Resuscitation and Emergency Cardiac Care, National Academy of Sciences - National Research Council Division of Medical Sciences   Committee on Emergency Medical Series (1974) Standards for cardiopulmonary resuscitation (CPR) and emergency cardiac care (ECC), V: medicolegal considerations and recommendations.   JAMA 227(Suppl):864-866
3. Rabkin MT, Gillerman G, Rice NR (1976) Orders not to resuscitate. N Engl J Med 295:364-66.
4. President's Commission for study of Ethical Problems in Medicine and Biomedical and Behavioral Research: Deciding to Forego Life-Sustaining   Treatment: A Report on The Ethical, Medical, and Legal Issues in Treatment Decisions. (1983) Washington, DC, U.S. Government Printing Office.   493-545
5. Standards for cardiopulmonary resuscitation (CPR) and emergency cardiac care (ECC). (1980) JAMA 244(Suppl):453-509
6. Vitelli CE, Cooper K, Rogatko A, Brennan MF (1991) Cardiopulmonary resuscitation and the patient with cancer.   J Clin Oncol 9:111-15
7. Miles SH, Cranford R, Shultz AL (1982) The do-not-resuscitate order in a teaching hospital:considerations and a suggested policy.   Ann Intern Med 96:660-64.
8. Bone RC, Rackow EC, Weg JG (1990) American College of Chest Physicians/Society for Critical Care Medicine Consensus Panel.   Ethical and moral guidelines for the initiation, continuation, and withdrawal of intensive care.   Chest 97:949-58.
9. Jonsson PV, McNamee M, Campion EW (1988) The 'Do Not Resuscitate' Order.   Arch Intern Med 148:2373-5.
10. Stolman CJ, Gregory JJ, Dunn D, Ripley B (1989) Evaluation of the do not resuscitate orders at   a community hospital.   Arch Intern Med 149:1851-56.
11. Evans AL, Brody BA (1985) The do-not-resuscitate order in teaching hospital.   JAMA 253:2236-39.
12. Schwartz DA, Reilly P (1986) The choice not to be resuscitated.   J Am Geriatr Soc 34:807-11.
13. Berowitz DR, Wilking SVB, Moskowitz MA (1991) Do-not-resuscitate orders at chronic care hospital.   J Am Geriatr Soc 39:472-76.
14. Bedell SE, Delbango TL (1984) Choices about cardiopulmonary resuscitation in the hospital.   N Engl J Med 310:1089-93.
15. Glesson K, Wise S (1990) The do-not-resuscitate order, still too little too late.   Arch Intern Med 150:1057-60.
16. Task Force on Ethics of the society of Critical Care Medicine (1989) Consensus report on the ethics of foregoing life-sustaining treatments in the critically ill.   Crit Care Med 18:1435-39.
17. Pijnenborg J, Maas PJ, Delden JJM, Looman CWN (1993) Life-terminating acts without explicit request of patient.   Lancet 341:1196-9.
18. Aarons EJ, Beeching NJ (1991) Survey of 'do not resuscitate' orders in a distinct general hospital.   Brit Med J 303:1504-6.

19. Asplund K, Britton M (1990) Do not resuscitate orders in Swedish medical wards. J Intern Med 228:139-145.
20. Delden JJM, Maas PJ, Pijnenborg L, Looman CWN (1993) Deciding not to resuscitate in Dutch hospitals. J Med Ethics 19:200-5.
21. Stanley DP, Reid DP (1989) Withholding cardiopulmonary resuscitation:one hospital's policy. Med J Aust 151:257-262.
22. The Appleton Consensus: suggested international guidelines for decisions to forego medical treatment (1989) J Med Ethics 15:129-136.
23. Stevens CA, Hassen R (1994) Management of death, dying and euthanasia:attitudes and practices of medical practitioners in South Australia. J Med Ethics 20:41-46.
24. Arai T, Namiki A, Amaha K, Shigematu A, Suzuki M, Kimura S, Miyazaki H, Nagaro T, Ogino K (1994) Response to a questionnaire on DNR order from 307 trustee members of Japanese medical societies. Masui 43:600-11. (in Japanese)
25. Arai T (1994) Informed consent on DNR-order. ICU & CCU 18:657-662. (in Japanese)
26. Fukaura A, Tazawa H, Sato I, Arai T, Sano H, Hirose T, Katura T, Mochizuki T, Sugihara S, Ohmori T, Horichi N, Nakajima H, Adachi M (1994) Survey of the physicians consciousness about D.N.R.(do not resuscitate) orders in treatment of patients with terminal lung cancers in Japan. J Jpn Soc Cancer Ther 29:1696-1708. (in Japanese)
27. Stern SG, Orlowski JP (1992) DNR or CPR-the choices is ours. Crit Care Med 20:1263-72.
28. Shapiro GR, Fefer I (1991) Do not resuscitate orders: the effect of the New York state law on cancer patients. Proc Annu Meet Am Soc Clin Oncol 10:A1143.
29. Uhlmann RF, Cassel CK, McDonald WJ (1984) Some treatment-withholding implications of no-code orders in an academic hospital. Crit Care Med 12:879-81.
30. Witte KL (1984) Variables present in patients who are either resuscitated or not resuscitated in a medical intensive care unit. Heart Lung 13:159-63.
31. Younger SJ (1987) Do-not resuscitate orders:no longer secret, but still a problem. Hasting Cent Rep 17:24-33.
32. Uhlman RF, McDonald J, Inui TS (1984) Epidemiology of no-code orders in an academic hospital. West J Med 140:114-116.
33. Wachter RM, Luce JM, Hearst N, Lo B (1989) Decisions about resuscitation: Inequities among patients with different diseases but similar prognosis. Ann Intern Med 111:325-332.
34. Lipton HL (1986) Do-not-resuscitate decisions in a community hospital: incidence, implications, and outcomes. JAMA 256:1164-1169.
35. The Prime Minister's Office, division of public information (1991) The public-opinion poll. Tokyo. The Ministry of Finance printing office 23(5):46-57. (in Japanese)
36. Sato I, Tazawa H, Fukaura A, Kasima N, Horichi N, Fujii H, Sugihara S, Mochizuki T, Katsura T, Nakajima H, Adachi M, Takahashi T (1994) The questionnaire about informing of cancer to the patients in Showa University Hospital. J Jpn Soc Cancer Ther 29:1677-1685. (in Japanese)
37. Murakami K, Haga T (1989) Cancer treatment in terminal stage. Jpn J Cancer Chemother 16:740-745 (in Japanese)
38. Murakami K, Haga T (1986) The protocol of informing cancer patients of their condition. Jpn J Cancer Chemother 13:2693-2698 (in Japanese)
39. Ishida T (1988) DNR-do not resuscitate. Kyukyuigaku 12:1103-1111 (in Japanese)
40. Tazawa H, Nakajima H, Ishihara J, Horichi N, Takahashi T, Sasaki Y (1986) Informed consent in patients with lung cancer. J Jpn Soc Cancer Ther 21:2454-2459 (in Japanese)
41. Tazawa H, Satoh I, Ishihara J, Ohmori T, Horichi N, Kashima N, Hiraizumi T, Takahashi T, Yamamoto M, Kasahara K, Sasaki Y (1990) Informed consent of the family in the chemotherapy for lung cancer. J Jpn Soc Cancer Ther 25:1448-1453 (in Japanese)
42. Teshima H, Kihara H, Ago Y, Kawamura H, Inoue T, Nagano H (1987) Terminal care for patients with lung cancer. Jpn J Thorac Dis 25:305-311 (in Japanese)

43. Fukaura A, Tazawa H, Nakajima H, Adachi M (1995) Do-not-resuscitate orders at a teaching hospital in Japan. N Engl J Med 333:805-808

44. Emanuel LL, Barry MJ, Stoeckle JD, Ettelson LM, Emanuel EJ (1991) Advanced directives for medical care. N Engl J Med 324:889-895

45. Sam M, Singer PA (1993) Canadian outpatients and advance directives. Can Med Assoc J 148:1497-1502

46. Brett As, McCullough LB (1986) When patients request specific interventions: defining the limits of the physician's obligation. N Engl J Med 315:1347-1351

47. Pellegriro ED (1992) Is truth telling to the patient a cultural artifact? JAMA 268:1734-1735

48. Fins JJ (1992) The patient self-determination act and patient-physician collaboration in New-York-state. New York State J Med 92:489-493

49. Fukaura A, Tazawa H, Sato I, Sugihara S, Mochizuki T, Hirose T, Ohmori T, Kasahara K, Nakajima H, Adachi M (1995) A prospective study of the inpatients' preferences on decision-making about medical problems and proxy. J Jpn Soc Cancer Ther 30:1333 (in Japanese)

50. Fukaura A, Arai T, Katsura T, Ohta S, Sato I, Horichi N, Kasahara K, Nakajima H, Adachi M (1996) Offering advance directive (personal medical directive). J Jpn Soc Cancer Ther 31:583 (in Japanese)

51. Emanuel LL, Emanuel EJ (1989) The medical directive a new comprehensive advance care document. JAMA 261:3288-3293

52. Brete AS (1991) Limitations of listing specitic medical interventions in advance directives. JAMA 266:825-828

53. The SUPPORT principal inrestigatons (1995) A controlled trial to improve care for seriously ill hospitalized patients. JAMA 274:1591-1598

54. Danis M, Southerland LI, Garrett JM, Smith JL, Hielema F (1991) A prospective study of advance directives for life-sustaining care. N Engl J Med 324:882-888

55. Schneiderman LT, Kronick R, Kaplan RM, Anderson JP. Langer RD (1992) Effects of offering advance directives on medical treatments and costs. Ann Inter Med 117:599-606

Ethical Dilemmas and Advance Directives in Japan

Atsushi Asai

Department of General Medicine and Clinical Epidemiology, Kyoto University School of Medicine, Kyoto University Hospital, Sakyo-ku, 606-01 Japan

SUMMARY. Recently a number of studies on clinical practices in Japan have been carried out. Researchers have conducted several clinical studies about ethical issues including life-sustaining treatment and advance directives. In this paper, I would like to review the studies published about these issues and also refer to the outcomes of two recent studies using a group interview with Japanese physicians and a nationwide survey. These results indicate that the general public, patients, and physicians in Japan think that advance directives would help to make medical care at the end of life more satisfactory. However, it has also been suggested that the wishes of patients or their advance directives are not always respected and that ethical decision making by Japanese physicians may depend on the situation and thus be inconsistent. It was also suggested that attitudes of physicians and a patient's family towards advance directives, life prolongation, and death with dignity can be possible barriers to implementing a competent patient's wishes or advance directives. Some physicians and family regard withholding or withdrawing of life support from a patient, even if according to the patient's wishes, as abandonment or killing. Furthermore, family's wishes to be at the bedside at the time of a patient's death seem to strongly affect the physician's decision about whether to perform cardiopulmonary resuscitation. We need to determine the importance of advance directives fro the Japanese and to find the best way to utilize such directives in Japanese clinical settings.

KEY WORDS: Advance directives, Life-sustaining treatment, Ethical dilemmas, Physician, Japan

1. CURRENT SITUATIONS IN REGARD TO LIFE-SUSTAINING TREATMENT AND ADVANCE DIRECTIVES IN JAPANESE CLINICAL SETTINGS

Life-sustaining treatment at the end of life and use of advance directives involve many ethical problems in Japan. In 1992, the Bioethics Council of the Japan Medical Association officially declared first that a physician should respect patient autonomy and written advance directives of a patient with terminal disease should be followed. When advance directives of an incompetent patient are not available, a family or a close friend can make a substitute judgment whether to discontinue life-sustaining treatment (1). An organization consisting of interdisciplinary intellectuals agreed with this recommendation (2). These recommendation indicates that physicians have to respect patient's wishes about medical care at the end-of-life. They also declared that there may be no legal problem not to resuscitate patients based on their wishes not to do so despite no explicit written law in Japan.

At this moment, more than 75,000 people have participated in the Japan Death with Dignity Association and had a living will (3). A recent public poll and a survey on patients showed that about 80% of respondents would want to discontinue life-prolonging interventions if they had advance directives an incurable, painful terminal disease. In addition, 31% of respondents considered it acceptable to discontinue all life-support (4, 5). A survey on inpatients in three hospitals in Japan revealed that 70% of 200 patients would want to die in home without aggressive life-prolonging interventions when they were terminally ill and two thirds of them would want sufficient pain control rather than life-prolongation (6). Younger people at the age of 20s to 30s shared the same opinions (7).

The recent public poll also revealed that 85% of 3030 respondents thought that usage of advance directive including a written document and explicit oral expression would be preferable and about half thought that advance directives should be legally regulated (4). The latest study published in 1997 revealed several important attitudes of Japanese public toward advance directives (8). More than 80% of 210 male subjects who visited two hospitals for their health check-ups knew the term "Living Will" and hoped to express their preferences toward medical care they will get in the future. More than 70% of them wanted to leave their preferences on treatment plan for incurable cancer, brain death, and persistent vegetative states as well as pain control. However, 80% answered that they would give a lot of leeway to surrogates to override their preferences and did not feel necessity for detailed and concrete directives. On the other hand, 40% of the respondents answered that they would observe advance directives that family members of the respondents leave and about half responded that it depends on contents the family member mentions. No one answered, however, that they would ignore the advance wishes that their family leave. A majority of physicians also considered patient's advance directives should be respected, while only 7% of them insisted life-prolongation regardless of advance directives (9). A recent survey on physicians working in university hospitals showed that 87% of physicians would follow patient's advance preferences about life prolongation and consult a designated surrogate if Japan had a law regulating advance directives and proxy. The main reasons to do so were to respect the patient's will and the right for medical care (10).

Barriers to respecting advance directives were pointed out. A study on nephrologists about termination of hemodialysis also suggested influence of family upon physician's decision. It showed that 88% of 72 Japanese physicians would withdraw hemodialysis from an incompetent patient if a patient left advance directives expressing his or her wishes to do so and family members agreed with his or her advance directives. While, less than one-fifth would discontinue hemodialysis from such a patient if family member insisted to continuing hemodialysis despite the patient's advance directives not to do so (11). Attitudes of Japanese physicians towards life-sustaining treatment could also be obstacles against the observance of advance directives. A comparative survey conducted in the US and Japan suggested that Japanese physicians tend to treat terminally-ill patients significantly more aggressively than Japanese-American physicians. Most Japanese physicians would recommend blood transfusion (74%), TPN (67%), vasopressor (61%) for terminally ill patients. Significantly fewer physicians would want these interventions for themselves. In addition, 36% of the responding Japanese physicians would override the patient's explicit wishes to discontinue life-support (12). Investigation on approximately 700 deceased patients in the past 10 years conducted in a general hospital provided us with clue of current situation of medical care at the end of life in Japan (13): 44% of them died of cancer. At the time of cardiopulmonary arrest, 14% underwent intubation, 6% had mechanical ventilation, and of the patients who died of cancer, 7% underwent intubation and 3% of underwent mechanical ventilation. Vasopressors were used for 64% and CPR were performed for 78% of all patients regardless of the underlying illness. These results are suggestive that both the general public and physicians seem to support use of advance directives for medical care to avoid unwanted medical intervention. They also suggest that patient's desires about death with dignity may not be guaranteed when family members or physicians insist life prolongation.

Despite these previous investigations, the current situation about how often advance directives are presented to physicians or to what extent they are respected are still unclear at present. To think though the impacts and benefits of advance directives in Japanese clinical settings, more reliable data about the actual situation is essential. Therefore, I would like to refer to the results of two recent studies conducted as parts of research projects regarding advance directives supported by the Grant for Scientific Research expenses for Health and Welfare Program; Funds for comprehensive research on Long Term chronic Disease (Renal Failure) in 1995 and 1996 (14, 15).

2. A GROUP INTERVIEW WITH JAPANESE PHYSICIANS REGARDING ADVANCE DIRECTIVES AND LIFE-SUSTAINING TREATMENT

Few studies have been undertaken to explore in depth the reasons why Japanese physicians treat terminally-ill patients aggressively and what affects the physicians' decisions so far in Japan. Our group interview was initiated to develop an in-depth understanding of Japanese physicians' attitudes toward life-sustaining treatment and advance directives. In December 1995, we conduct a focus group interview with 7 Japanese physicians. The interview inquired as to the physicians' attitudes toward advance directives and possible barriers in using them in the clinical setting. A qualitative study design and analysis were employed to gain an in-depth understanding of attitudes and rationales in Japan regarding medical care at the end of life. The complete record of the interview has been published elsewhere (16).

The physicians were recruited from 6 different medical institutions; all were male, ranging in age from 31 to 41 years old. All were internists who treat patients with cancer and other serious diseases in daily practice. Analysis revealed that physicians and patients' family members usually make decisions about life-sustaining treatment, while the patients' wishes are unavailable or not taken into account. Both physicians and family members tend to consider withholding or withdrawing life-sustaining treatment as abandonment or even killing. Family members' desire to be at the bedside at the time of death seems to be the strongest reason to start cardiopulmonary resuscitation and continue it until patients' family members arrive. No participant held the belief that the end of life should be prolonged. All physicians participating in our study regarded advance directives that provide patients' wishes about life-sustaining treatment desirable. All expressed concern, however, that it would be difficult to forgo or discontinue life support based on a patient's advance directives, particularly when the patient's family opposes the directives. Despite the official statement of the Japan Medical Association, the physicians feared family lawsuits or accusations of killing the patient. The findings suggest that some Japanese physicians may regard withholding and withdrawing life-sustaining treatment as ethically or legally unacceptable, rather than regarding these measures as a means to a peaceful death with dignity.

3. A NATIONAL SURVEY REGARDING ETHICAL DILEMMAS AND ADVANCE DIRECTIVES IN JAPANESE CLINICAL SETTINGS

Based on the outcomes gained from the group interview mentioned in the previous section, we designed a nationwide survey on Japanese physicians to reveal their experiences of and attitudes toward life-sustaining treatment and advance directives in a quantitative form. We asked the participants about what kind of ethical dilemmas they are experiencing in everyday basis using an open-ended question. The questionnaire asked about their experience in regard to wishes or advance directives about unwanted medical intervention presented by their patients, the rate of observing or overriding these, and the occurrence of cardiopulmonary resuscitation for arrested terminal patients in order to enable their family to be at the bedside at the time of patient's cardiac death (CPR for patient's family). We defined advance directives as wishes regarding unwanted medical intervention presented in advance by a competent patient to guide future medical care when the patient becomes incompetent. It includes oral advance directives and a document such as a living will. Since there are currently no legal regulations about advance directives in Japan, we did not limit it to written documents only.

Ethical dilemmas in clinical settings (15)

More than 300 physicians participated in the survey and three-fourths of them answered that they were perplexed by ethical dilemmas in medical decisions concerning the end of life. Only 3% responded that they were never perplexed by such dilemmas. Approximately 80% described one or more the most perplexing ethical dilemmas that they experiences in their practice. A total of 386 dilemmas were described as the most perplexing.

Of 267 respondents who described ethical dilemmas, 68% of the respondents reported dilemmas with regard to life-sustaining treatment. They included indication of cardiopulmonary resuscitation (CPR) for a terminal patient, ethical implication of withdrawal of life support from them, and whether mechanical ventilation should be provided with a terminal patient with severe respiratory failure. Decisions whether to initiate or terminate other interventions including hemodialysis, blood transfusion, total parenteral nutrition, antibiotics were also mentioned. Seventeen- percent of them reported dilemmas with regard to problems involving patient's family. Among them, how to deal with disagreement in wishes for medical care between patient and his or her family presented the commonest ethical problems. Family's refusal or demand to performing life-sustaining treatment for their patient were also reported. Disagreement among family members regarding plan of patient's care were also reported. About 15% reported dilemmas with regard to patient's refusal or demand of medical care. Patient's request to have all possible interventions that are considered medically futile, and refusal to effective treatment were mentioned. Some reported that they experienced difficulty to make decisions because no patient's wishes for terminal care were available. thirteen-percent of the respondents reported dilemmas with regard to truth telling to a terminal cancer patient, including requests of patient's family not to inform a true diagnosis and prognosis to patients and whether to inform a patient of the exact prognosis of the terminal illness. Some respondents experienced the difficulty to take care of a terminal patient who was unaware of their destiny.

Responses in the open ended question revealed various ethical problems in Japanese clinical settings. The followings includes concrete questions the respondent had. Many respondents questioned whether CPR should be performed for a terminal patient and not sure if it is necessary. Some other concerned CPR for the aged and the demented. Some reported that they perform CPR for a terminal patient although they believe that we should not do it. Resuscitating a cardiac arrested patient with terminal cancer for the sake of patient's family is also common problem. Some had a policy not to perform CPR for a terminal patient unless patient's family members are not at the bedside at the time of death. Many questioned if it is ethically proper to perform CPR for a terminal patient because of the request of patient' family.

An ethical question regarding withholding of life support of a terminal or unconscious patient is also one of major problems. Many questioned their dilemmas like the following: "Should a physician aggressively treat a demented patient who is totally dependent and bed-ridden?," "There is a question if it is appropriate to use very expensive treatment for a terminal patient", "Is it appropriate to sustain the life of a patient with PVS in the long interval," " Is it appropriate for a physician to go aggressive medical intervention for old comatose patient?," or "Should we continue hemodialysis for severely demented patients?" Questions regarding indication of various medical interventions are also regarded by the respondents as perplexing dilemmas. Mechanical ventilation for a terminal cancer patient who has serious pneumonia or for a patient who has no chance of recovery, blood transfusion for a patient who is bleeding from terminal cancer, hyperalimetation for irreversibly unconscious cancer patients, or hemodialysis for a terminal patient with renal failure were mentioned. Whether discontinuation of life-sustaining treatment is ethically permissive or not was also one of the perplexing ethical dilemmas the respondents raised. They asked, "When should we extubate from a moribund patient or when should we withdraw antibiotics or blood transfusion from a terminal patient?" At the same time, how to deal with patient's refusal of life-sustaining treatment was mentioned as problematic. Patient's refusal of having fluid replacement for dehydration made the respondents feel uncomfortable to decide what to do.

Experiences regarding Advance Directives   (15)

The questionnaire asked the respondents about advance directives presented by their patients and its contents. First of all, approximately 40% of the respondents had been presented advance directives by their patients, and 10% of the patients whom the respondents had cared for presented them with them.

Medical situations patients referred to in their advance directives included no chance of recovery, irreversible consciousness disturbance, suffering from intractable pain, persistent respiratory distress, and cardiopulmonary arrest. Unwanted medical interventions mentioned by patients included cardiopulmonary resuscitation, life-prolonging acts in general, mechanical ventilation and blood transfusion . others reported advance directives that asked for sufficient palliative care. CPR was by far the most frequent unwanted intervention indicated in the advance directives, and total parenteral nutrition and intravenous fluid were mentioned as unwanted life-prolonging acts. Patient's wishes that all medical intervention should be terminated at a certain point were also expressed in the advance directives.

About one-third of the respondents whose patients presented them with advance directives followed all of them, half followed more than half, and less than 10% answered that they followed less than one-fourth. Among the reported reasons to follow or override a patient's advance directives, the most frequent reason for following a patient's advance directives was the respondent's belief that a patient's rights and wishes in medical care should be respected. This was followed by the respondents' judgment that the patient's QOL was poor and the perception that life-sustaining treatment was futile. On the other hand, the reasons for overriding advance directives varied and they included family wishes to sustain a patient's life, high possibility of recovery, and absence of the patient's family at the bedside. Most respondents regarded advance directives useful for the provision of care for their terminal patients. Respondents were asked about their experience with CPR for arrested terminal patients in order to enable their family to be at the bedside at the time of the death (CPR for patient's family). Only 4% of the respondents had never performed CPR for patient's family, while 7% performed it in all cases. Approximately half of them performed it for one-fourth of their cases, one-fourth of them for half, and one-fifth of them for three-fourths.

DISCUSSION

I have reviewed several published studies and summarized two recent investigations conducted by us, using a group interview and a nationwide survey in regard to life-sustaining treatment and advance directives. The studies reviewed suggest that the general public, patients, and physicians in Japan think that advance directives would help to make medical care at the end of life more satisfactory. However, family wishes to prolong the life of the terminally ill at any cost and physicians' preference to treat such patients aggressively have been pointed out as possible obstacles to implementing a patient's advance directives.

The results of two fact finding studies conducted in 1995 and 1996 have added some new information of the current situations with regard to medical decisions concerning the end of life and advance directives, and also suggested possible barriers to implementing them (15). First, Japanese physicians face a variety of perplexing ethical dilemmas; they include CPR for the terminally ill, decision about withholding and/or withdrawing life-prolonging interventions, disagreement among parties involved in regard to planning patient care, and so on. This means that Japanese physicians have been experiencing the common dilemmas in clinical settings identified and discussed in many other countries (16-22).

Some of the latest clinical studies conducted in Japan confirmed this situation. A survey on medical residents in Japan reveals that half of the respondents reported that they were sometimes perplexed by ethical problems involved in patient care, 22% often, and 11% responded that they were perplexed by ethical problems very frequently in everyday practice. Only 16% of the respondents reported they were rarely or never perplexed by such problems. On average, the respondents estimated that one-third of the patient care they were in charge of involved ethical problems. The ethical problems that the residents reported to be confronted with most frequently were medical decisions concerning the end of life: 43% of 113 residents were perplexed by such problems. The next most common problems were truth telling (37%) and how to obtain valid informed consent (12%) (23). Another study conducted in a general medicine ward at a university hospital shows that ethical dilemmas frequently identified included refusal of or unnecessary requests for diagnostic procedures or treatment by patients, issues concerning truth-telling to patients with a serious illness, and disagreement regarding plans for patient care between patients' family and physicians in charge (24).

Second, our study shows that approximately 40% of Japanese physicians who are mainly taking care of cancer patients have been presented advance directives by their patients and that, on average, 10% of the patients that our respondents encountered in their practice gave them their advance directives. Although it is unlikely that these results are representative of the present overall situation in regard to advance directives in Japan, these results should be regarded as highly significant, given the situation where there are currently no legal regulations, practical guidelines, or agreement about advance directives in clinical settings. Our results, therefore, indicate the need to consider the meaning and role of advance directives in Japan.

Third, our studies suggest that patients' advance directives may not be respected in all cases. Only one-third of the respondents whose patients presented them with advance directives followed all of them. Our interview and survey provided us with new insights into the reasons why some physicians are reluctant to observe such instructions. 1) Some patients' family members want to be at the bedside at the time of a patient's death, and some physicians agree that this is desirable. Some physicians might think that CPR is a kind of ritual that they have to perform at the time of the patient death. 2) A physician and a patient's family may regard withholding or discontinuing life-prolonging interventions as abandonment or even murder, rather than death with dignity. Such considerations would constitute significant barriers to implementing patient's advance wishes to avoid unwanted medical intervention.

In summary, the general public, patients, and physicians in Japan think that advance directives would help for making medical care at the end of life more satisfactory. On the other hand, there are many obstacles to utilizing such directives in clinical settings. The current situation regarding life-sustaining treatment and advance directives is still chaotic and decisions are inconsistent. Ethical decisions made by Japanese physicians may be situation-bound and be under strongly influenced by the patient's family. We need to determine the importance of advance directives and find the best way to implement them in Japanese clinical settings.

REFERENCES

1: The Bioethical Committee for Japanese Medical Association (1992) Special report about "What physicians faced with patients with terminal illness should do." J Jpn Med Association 107: 1209-17 (In Japanese)
2: Special report about Death and Medicine: Death with Dignity (1994) Special Committee for Death and Medicine. Nihon Gakujutsu Kaigi (In Japanese)
3. Sakamoto T, Kitazawa K (1996) Confronted with "death." Nikkei Medical 10; 46-60 (In Japanese)
4. Report from a survey on Japanese general public regarding their
preferences towards terminal care (1994) Tokyo: Division of Public Policy,
Ministry of Health and Welfare (In Japanese)
5. Takuchi Y, Yazawa Y, Sakakibara Y, Tanaka R (1995) A survey on the aged regarding terminal care. Rojin Kango. 26; 160 (In Japanese)
6. Kai I, Ohi G, Yano E, Kobayashi Y, Miyata T, Niino N, Naka K (1993) Comminication between patients and physicians about
terminal care: A survey in Japan. SSM 36; 1151-1159
7. Kono F, Sakashita T, and Kihara N (1995) A survey regarding death and
terminal care. Nihon Kango Kenkyu-Kan Zasshi 18; 98(In Japanese)
8. Akabayashi A, Kai I, Iton K, Tsukui K (1997) The acceptability of advance directives in Japanese society - A questionnaire study for healthy heople in the physical check-up settings. JJAB 7;31-40 (In Japanese)
9. The Bioethical Committee for Japanese Medical Association (1994) Report regarding informed consent. J Jpn Med Association (Nihon Ishika Zashi) 103; 515-528 (In Japanese)
10. Macer D, Hosaka T, Nimura Y, Umeno T, Wakai K (1996) Attitudes of university doctors to the use of advance directives, euthanasia and bioethics in Japan. EJAIB 6; 63-69
11. Sehgal AR, Weisheit C, Miura Y, Butzlaff M, Kielstein R, Taguchi Y (1996) Advance directives and withdrawal of dialysis in the United States, Germany, and Japan. JAMA 276; 1652-1656.
12. Asai A, Fukuhara S, Lo B (1995) Attitudes of Japanese and Japanese-American physicians towards life-sustaining treatment. Lancet 346; 356-359
13. Yoshimoto M, Senga K, Kondo F (1995) Current situation of terminal care in a hospital. Shi No Rinsho 18; 218 (In Japanese)
14. Asai A, Inoshita O, Fukuhara S, Miura Y, Tanabe N,Matsumuta S (1995) A study regarding advance directives. Report of research projects supported by the Grant for Scientific Research expenses for Health and Welfare Program; Funds for comprehensive research on Long Term chronic Disease (Renal Failure) p 9-12.
15. Miura Y, Asai A, Fukuhara S, Tanabe N, Kurihara N (1996) A study regarding advance directives. Report of research projects supported by the Grant for Scientific Research expenses for Health and Welfare Program; Funds for comprehensive research on Long Term chronic Disease (Renal Failure) p 7-11.
16. Asai A, Fukuhara S, Inoshita O, Miura Y, Tanabe T, Kurokawa K (1997) Medical decisions concerning the end of life: A discussion with Japanese physicians. Journal of Medical Ethics In Press
17. Singer PA (1994) Disease-specific advance directices. Lancet 344; 594 - 596
18. Gordon M, Singer PA (1995) Decisions and care at the end of life. Lancet 346; 163 - 165
19. Morrison RS, Olson E, Mertz KR, Meier DE (1996) The inaccessibility of advance directives on transfer from ambulatoru to acute care settings. JAMA 274: 478 - 482

20. Grubb AG, Walsh P. Lambe N, Murrells T, Robinson S (1996) Survey of British clinicians' views on management of patients in perisitent vegetative state. Lancet 348; 35 - 40

21. Lo B (1995) Resolving ethical dilemmas : a guide for clinicians. Baltimore: Williams and Wilkins

22. Thomsen O, Wulff HR, Martin A, Singer PA (1993) What gastroenterologists in Europe tell cancer patients? Lancet 341; 473 - 476

23. Asai A, Kishino M, Fukui T, Masano T (1997) Postgraduate education in medical ethics in Japan. Medical Education In press

24. Asai A, Yamamoto W, T Fukui (1997) What ethical dilemmas are Japanese physicians faced with? EJAIB In press

Session Summary

Ethics in Palliative Medicine

Tetsuro Shimizu[1]

[1]Faculty of Arts and Letters, Tohoku University, Kawauchi, Aoba-ku, Sendai 980-8576 Japan

In this session we were concerned with ethical issues that are involved in Palliative Medicine. Before the three speakers' presentations, Professor Stephen C. Schimpff, a chairperson of the session, gave introductory remarks. He discussed Palliative Medicine as an exemplar of the new paradigm for medicine, i.e. holistic care, in comparison with the curative model that has been predominant. The significant difference between the two models lies in the value to which each model assigns priority, i.e., curative attitude of combatting disease vs. holistic medicine's care for the patient as a human being, etc. On the basis of Dr. Schimpff's presentation, we can also recognize how research into the ethical aspects of palliative medicine is related to its conception with respect to the new paradigm, for the change of priority of values results in a certain shift of ethical judgements as well.

The first speaker, Dr. Geert H. Blijham, reported the basic facts concerning euthanasia and physician-assisted suicide in the Netherlands, including the fact that the main reason for requesting euthanasia or physician assisted suicide is not the unbearable pain but the unrecoverable lack of human dignity caused by the disease. He concluded that euthanasia does not exclude good palliative care nor should good palliative care exclude euthanasia. The question was raised of how to distinguish the patient's request for euthanasia or physician-assisted suicide as an autonomous self-determination that could be granted from the expression of a spiritual problem in the patient that should be cared for. The speaker replied, first, that the solution of how to care for patients in the last four or five weeks of their life is certainly different from country to country depending on the culture or tradition, and, secondly, that listening to patients is important. For patients in personal communication with the physician often express their negative reply to the existential question concerning the meaning of the last four weeks of their life, while there can also be a positive reply depending on the patients' belief systems or religious backgrounds. Additional comments included the fact that the discussion concerning the possibility of euthanasia in terms of palliative medicine has started also in other countries, including the U.S. and Belgium, and the observation that people's attitudes sometimes depend on their religious backgrounds, e.g., a reason of allowing euthanasia is derived from a belief in life after death.

The second speaker, Dr. Asato Fukaura, reported the introduction of a standardized do-not-resuscitate order form at his university hospital and its effectiveness in lessening the cases of futile cardiopulmonary resuscitation in patients dying of lung cancer. He concluded that the introduction of do-not-resuscitate order forms and personal medical directives are useful for the patient's interest. A participant commented that the notification of disease, which the patient needs for being able to give do-not-resuscitate order appropriately, does not seem sufficient. Then, physicians' and families' negative attitudes towards the notification in Japan became the subject of discussion, including the claim that the average rate of notification of cancer must be much higher in many Japanese hospitals today than the speaker's data suggests is the case for his hospital. Nevertheless, the report remains significant in that it represents a model of efforts to promote the new paradigm of medicine in hospitals where the curative model is still predominant.

The last speaker, Dr. Atsushi Asai, reported the extent to which, among Japanese physicians, the patient's wishes, including advance directives, are taken into consideration in medical decisions concerning the end of life. He showed that the main reason for following advance directives is the patients' right to determine their own medical care, while the main reason for overriding them is the family's wishes to prolong life, which seemed to be one of the biggest barriers to implementing a competent patient's advance directives towards the end of life. Concerning the report it was discussed that the family's influence in medical decisions in Japan seems to be somewhat different from that in western countries, but beyond the cultural difference the patient's self-determination, and not the family's will, should have priority. In order to avoid misunderstanding, it should be noted that also the family, which is involved in the palliative medicine, should be appropriately cared for with respect to the quality of life, and again the patient's good relationship with the family improves the patient's quality of life, so that it is better if the family can be brought to agree with the patient, and the medical staff has to try to bring about harmony between them. Nevertheless, it never means that they are allowed to prioritize the family's will over the patient's own will.

Through the three reports along with the introductory remarks and discussions, the central points of the ethical issues in palliative medicine became apparent. Dr. Schimpff concluded that the physician has to have a truthful relationship with patients and to recognize their personal autonomy, so that the physician has to ask them what their needs are and not to put the physician's own values or beliefs over those of the patients. Those conclusions are consistent with the concept of the holistic approach to medical care he referred to in his introductory remarks.

What I would like to have added to the conclusions is as follows. There are two main aspects of ethical issues; first, the choice of value among diverse values, which are sometimes incompatible with each other, and, secondly, the process of decision making, which consists mainly of the choice of value. Euthanasia is thought, at least by people with a positive attitude towards it, to be the choice of death which is more valuable in some cases than a life of suffering, and the choice will never be granted if not based on the patient's autonomous determination. Do-not-resuscitate orders as well as advance directives concern the process of decision making in terms of the patient's self-determination, by which the patient determines the priority among diverse values.

Thus the first aspect concerns the goodness that is aimed at *by* the chosen medical activities, while the second aspect has to do with the goodness *in* the process of choosing medical activities. The former goodness should be chosen by the patient, and the latter lies only in the fact that the patient autonomously chooses the former. Consequently the medical staff should support the competent patient being able to make autonomous decisions through trustful communication with the patient (and with the family as well) and should agree with the patient's choice that the medical staff recognizes as reasonable and consistent. This implies the process of shared decision making and is one of the most important ethical prescriptions to the medical staff. As to the case of the patient's incompetency, an ethical prescription could be that the medical staff as well as the family should behave as advocates of the patient, but there was not enough discussion in the present session to examine it in detail.

Session V

Health Economics in Palliative Medicine

Chairpersons:
Ronald Feld and Shigeaki Yoshida

HEALTH ECONOMICS OF PALLIATIVE THERAPY

Smith, TJ [1]

[1]Faculty Scholar, *Project on Death in America*, Open Society, New York; Associate Professor of Medicine; Massey Cancer Center; Virginia Commonwealth University/Medical College of Virginia, Richmond, Virginia, U.S.A. 23298-0037.

SUMMARY. Cancer care is expensive due to increasing age, more cancer cases, increased demand for treatment, and new expensive technologies. We must use our the limited resources wisely so that we can provide both curative and palliative care. Since palliative therapy does not cure cancer or gain years of life, it often does not have a measurable cost-effectiveness ratio. Cost-utility ratios, which add the improvement in health to the life years gained, may not change much with palliative therapy. The improvements in health state are too small, or are lost because the impact of the disease is so large. Only a few studies have assessed the economics of palliative therapy. The major areas of interest include palliative chemotherapy vs. best supportive care; supportive care for cancer symptoms; the process and structure of care; follow up; and hospice care. Chemotherapy for Stage III and IV non-small cell lung cancer, mitoxantrone for prostate cancer, and chemotherapy for gastrointestinal cancer have acceptable cost-effectiveness ratios. There are many ways to save money and improve supportive care for infections, nausea, and pain. Hospice care gives care equal to regular care, but will save only 3%. Coordination of care will not improve the clinical outcomes of dying patients, but will save 40% of costs. The cost of palliative therapy is so small, and the benefits so large, that it should always be included in a list of approved treatments.

KEY WORDS: Health economics, cancer, palliative therapy

INTRODUCTION

Health care spending and health care quality in the United States are major problems. Cancer care costs have risen from $35 billion in 1990 [1] to $40 billion in 1994 [2] to $50 billion by 1996 [3]. There is concern that we may be spending too much on high technology care for the elderly, since nearly one third of all Medicare spending is on patients in their last year of life [4,5]. This may be medically appropriate care, but those dollars cannot be spent on preventive services or chronic disease conditions for the same population [6]. The allocation of health care dollars is a "political nightmare" due to increased demands for care from an educated elderly population, more elderly long term survivors, new and expensive technologies, new diseases like acquired immunodeficiency syndrome, and demands for cost cutting [7,8].

Care given to patients in their last phase of life could improve in quality. The SUPPORT study showed that half of all dying patients had unnecessary pain and suffering in their final days of life while in the hospital [9]. In the outpatient setting, nearly half of the patients suffer unnecessary pain even when cared for by oncologists or academic oncologists [10]. The care given to cancer given to cancer patients in general can be improved. For breast cancer, substantial practice variation by geographic region has been documented with some states having five times the number of mastectomies versus the preferred method of breast conserving lumpectomy and radiation [11,12]. Hillner et al documented substantial under use of adjuvant therapy [13]; and under use of surveillance mammography in patients after breast cancer treatment, with about 20% having no follow up mammogram within two years [14]. Our group has documented substantial under-use of thoracotomy in the elderly with lung cancer compared to younger patients [15], and similar patterns in prostate cancer [16]. There appears to be significant (5%) overall survival advantage to care given at a cancer specialty center for breast cancer, rather than at community hospitals [17,18]; better survival for testicular cancer patients treated at specialist centers [19]; and better survival and fewer complications for ovarian cancer surgery performed by specialist gynecologic oncologists rather than general surgeons or gynecologists [20]. It is clear that the process of care may not be optimal for all patients.

Table 1 lists the important questions to be asked.

Table 1. Types of studies of health and service research studies

Type of study	Question posed
Type of care: chemotherapy vs. best or other types of supportive care chemotherapy	Does chemotherapy save money compared to best supportive care, when all costs are considered?
The site of service	Is home vs. hospitals more effective and less costly?
Structural and process changes in care	Can costs of care be reduced by changes in how it is delivered? e.g. by coordination or at home?
Hospice vs. non hospice	Does hospice improve quality of life or reduce costs of care?
Advanced directives and Do Not Resuscitate Orders	Do advanced directives influence medical treatment decisions or change costs?

METHODS

I reviewed Medline from 1980 to 1997 for relevant articles, and did selected searches within bibliographies.

RESULTS

Data Available to Decision Makers

It is important to organize data in a way useful to decision makers. Most cancer treatment decisions are helped by presenting clinical and cost information side by side. The usual types of cost studies are shown in Table 2.

Table 2. Ways to present results clinical and cost studies to decision-makers

Type of study	Advantages and Disadvantages
Clinical outcomes only	Ignores costs. Ex - Easy to choose among clearly superior therapies such as cisplatin for testicular cancer; harder among all others that give lesser benefits at high costs.
Cost only, e.g costs of treating febrile neutropenia	Ignores clinical outcomes. Does not help decision makers choose among clinical strategies. Ex - The cost of colony stimulating factor (CSF) mobilization of stem cells may be higher than that of bone marrow collection, but it saves money later by reducing hospital stay.
Costs and clinical outcomes together	
Cost-minimization	Assumes that two strategies are equal; lowest cost strategy is preferred
Cost-effectiveness	Compares two strategies; assigns $ per additional year of life (LY) saved by strategy. Ex - At present, CSF's have not improved survival, so cost must be lower for therapy to be cost-effective.
Cost-utility	Compares two strategies; assigns $ per additional year of life (LY) saved by strategy, then estimates the quality of that benefit in $/quality adjusted (QALY). Ex - No data show significant improvement in quality of life or utilities in patients who have received CSFs, so unlikely to have major impact.
Cost-benefit	Compares two strategies but converts the clinical benefits to money, e.g. a year of life is worth $100,000. Possible but rarely done due to difficulty in assigning $ value to benefit; requires assigning a value to human life

Chemotherapy versus best supportive care

These strategies are often considered opposite, when both are trying to help the patient. Chemotherapy for incurable solid tumors may be helpful for symptom relief or to prolong survival. The key is to make the switch to supportive care while resources and good quality tin.e are still available [21]. The American Society of Clinical Oncology has outlined appropriate outcomes that justify therapy in cancer patients listed in Table 3 [22]. These justifications for treatment apply to both palliative care and chemotherapy.

Table 3. American Society of Clinical Oncology Outcomes that justify diagnostic tests or treatments [22]

Outcomes that justify use	Outcomes that do not justify use
Improved overall survival	Earlier knowledge about recurrence
Improved disease free survival	
Better quality of life	Unproven hope of better care or palliation
Less toxicity	
Improved cost-effectiveness	Cost alone

The Expert Panel could not define a minimum amount of benefit required to justify treatment, but a least some benefit in symptoms or disease control was required.

It is critical to remember that patients may view benefit and toxicity in ways very different from their health care providers Dying patients would undergo almost any treatment toxicity for a 1% chance of short term survival, while their doctors and nurses would not [23]. A study of palliative radiotherapy for brain tumor patients showed little survival and modest functional benefit, and a substantial decrement in intellectual function, but most patients and families would still want it [24,25].

Cost effectiveness as an outcome

The funding of treatments based on cost-effectiveness ratios is possible [26]. Laupacis and colleagues [27] in Canada have proposed this funding level: 1) treatments that clearly work and are less expensive be adopted readily; 2) those with cost-effectiveness ratios <$20,000 per additional year of life (LY) gained be accepted with the recognition that they cost additional resources; 3) that treatments with cost effectiveness ratios $20,000-$100,000/LY be examined on a case by case basis with caution; 4) and that treatments with cost effectiveness ratios of >$100,000/LY be rejected. This system is valid in a system where all resources are shared equally; it is not clear how this system applies to other health care systems where resources may not be shared [28]. Alternatively, patients might be allowed to purchase additional insurance for expensive treatments, or pay for them out of pocket. In the United States, there has been no accepted answer but most authorities have agreed on an implicitly defined benchmark of $35,000-$50,000 per year of life saved [26].

Disease Examples: Lung, Gastrointestinal, Prostate, Breast Cancer, and Leukemia

It is possible to give chemotherapy and either save money, or have a cost effectiveness within accepted limits as shown in Table 4. Patient treated with chemotherapy for non small cell lung cancer have a small benefit, estimated at 2-4 months in most series [29,30], and symptom relief in up to 60% [31]. Both the American Society of Clinical Oncology [32] and Ontario government [33] recommend consideration of chemotherapy for suitable patients. Jaakimainen et al found that chemotherapy actually saved disease management costs compared to best supportive care by preventing hospitalizations late in the disease course. The cost effectiveness ratios ranged from $-8,000 (cost saving) to $+20,000 Canadian for each additional year of life [34]. Smith and colleagues found that chemotherapy with cisplatin and vinorelbine, compared to vinorelbine alone or cisplatin and vindesine, added substantial clinical benefit [35] at a reasonable cost effectiveness of $15,000-$17,000 per year of life [36]. Given the benefit and low cost of the drugs, vinorelbine and cisplatin compared to best supportive care would give results similar to those of Jaakimainen and colleagues [34]. Evans and colleagues used decision analysis to show that chemotherapy in combination with radiation and/or surgery for Stage IIIA or IIIB disease, in comparison to treatment without chemotherapy would improve survival at a cost of $3,348 to $14,958 Canadian per year of life saved [37]. The model showed benefit at a reasonable cost under all situations of reasonable clinical efficacy. The chemotherapy treatments fit existing monetary guidelines for use[38,39].

Gastrointestinal patients were randomized to first line chemotherapy vs. best supportive care that could include later chemotherapy for symptom control [40]. For the whole group, chemotherapy enhanced survival by about 5 months at a cost of about $20,000 per year of life gained, within accepted bounds [26]. For subsets of types of cancer, such as gastric cancer, the treatment was effective at a reasonable cost. For most other subsets, the patient numbers were too small to draw meaningful conclusions about either clinical effect or cost-effectiveness.

In the only prostate cancer study, mitoxantrone added a small clinical benefit in terms of pain relief and symptom control in 23 of 80 patients, lasting for 6 more months than prednisone alone, for several months, but did not alter survival when compared to prednisone alone [41]. Although initial drug costs were higher, total disease costs were lower in the group that received mitoxantrone as initial treatment [42], so good chemotherapy palliation could be accomplished at no additional cost to society.

Studies on the effectiveness or cost effectiveness of chemotherapy for metastatic breast cancer compared to best supportive care have not been reported. Hospitalization accounts for the majority of costs, while chemotherapy has been a relatively trivial cost [43]. In the only available study of comparative treatment, Hillner et al compared best standard chemotherapy to high dose chemotherapy (HDC) with a stem cell transplant [44]. HDC added about six months at a cost effectiveness ratio of $116,000 per year of life gained. Although not routinely considered palliative care, HDC is commonly used for incurable metastatic disease, and in the one randomized controlled trial doubled overall survival from 10.4 to 20.8 months although it did not appear to produce a long term survival plateau [45].

Acute myelogenous leukemia chemotherapy cost more than supportive care and certain death, and allogeneic transplant was even more effective. The transplant survival benefit 48% versus 21% at 5 years was sufficient to offset higher costs of treatment and make the cost-effectiveness ratio about $18,000/LY [46].

Table 4. Chemotherapy vs. Best supportive care or alternative treatments

Topic	Conclusion
Lung cancer	
Chemotherapy vs. best supportive care in non-small cell lung cancer [34]	Chemotherapy gained 8-13 weeks compared to best supportive care. Chemotherapy generally saved money for the province of Ontario, from a savings of $8,000 Can to additional cost of $20,000 depending on assumptions.
Combined modality including chemotherapy vs. Radiation or surgery for Stage III non-small cell lung cancer [37-39]	Chemotherapy in combination with radiation or surgery adds clinical benefit; for chemotherapy plus radiation one and five-year survival is increased from 40 to 54% and 6 to 17%, for instance. The addition of chemotherapy for IIIA patients added cost of $$15,866, and addition of chemotherapy to IIIB patients added $8,912. The cost year of life gained was well within accepted bounds at $3,348 to $14,958 Canadian.
Alternating chemotherapy for small cell lung cancer [47]	The alternating chemotherapy arm cost more, but because it was more effective, the marginal cost effectiveness was only $4,560/LY.
Gastrointestinal cancer	
Chemotherapy vs. Best supportive care followed by chemotherapy for GI cancer patients [40]	Chemotherapy added 5 months median survival if given early rather than late, with symptom palliation for 4 months. The additional cost of about $20,000/life year was within accepted bounds.
Prostate cancer	
Palliative chemotherapy with mitoxantrone plus prednisone vs. prednisone [41,42]	Mitoxantrone did not improve survival, but improved quality of life as measured by several indices, and the mitoxantrone strategy cost less than prednisone supportive care.
Breast cancer	
High dose chemotherapy for limited metastatic disease vs. standard chemotherapy [44]	High dose chemotherapy added 6 months at a cost of $58,000, or $116,000/LY; this is palliative care as this treatment has not been shown to be curative.
Other	
Acute myelogenous leukemia [46]	Chemotherapy, compared to supportive care, added additional cost but the cost effectiveness was $18,000/LY, within acceptable limits.

Modified from Smith et al [26].

Site of service

The limited studies are shown in Table 5. Home narcotic infusions had higher drug equipment, and nursing costs, but lower total costs due to less hospital costs [48]. Outpatient administration of chemotherapy was less expensive than inpatient administration [49]. There is no only one study that compares home chemotherapy to outpatient chemotherapy [50]. The program was well-accepted with only two of 424 patients electing to discontinue home treatment. Home chemotherapy was safe, and the average cost was $50 compared to $116 in hospital, with equal total costs.

Table 5. Site of service

Topic	Conclusion
Narcotics [48]	Narcotics at home per diem costs were higher for home patients, but total costs were lower with equivalent palliation
Inpatient or outpatient chemotherapy [49]	Outpatient administration was less expensive, $184 vs. 223 in US$.
Home or inpatient/clinic chemotherapy [50]	Home chemotherapy was safe, well accepted, and cost less per treatment

Changes in process or structure of care

Changes in disease management have shown some dramatic improvements but the data may be proprietary and not available. For instance, coordinated disease management by an expert team expanded home care services for AIDS patients by 600% but decreased total costs by nearly 50% (unpublished data, First Boston Corporation.) Similar results were seen in the disease management of congestive heart failure. The available studies are shown in Table 6.

Coordinated care offers many advantages for terminally ill cancer patients. The Medicare Hospice Benefit requires nurse coordination, team management, easy access to low per diem hospital beds for respite or temporary care, and expanded drug coverage [51,52]. Adding a nurse coordinator for terminally ill patients in England did not change any disease outcomes; patients still died, and most still had some unrelieved symptoms, but patient and family satisfaction was helped slightly [53]. The total costs were reduced from £8814 to £4414 for a cost savings of 41% in almost all conditions [54]. The savings came from decreased hospital days.

Most patients prefer to die at home. Making nursing care available was associated with more patients dying at home [55].

A pain management system-wide intervention with enhanced institutional education programs, a highly visible respected consultative team, and a pain resource center for nurses and families was associated with a decrease in admissions and re-admissions for pain control [56]. The study was not randomized, and could not account for other significant changes such as the growth of managed care with restricted admission policies. However, the conclusion must be that this is better pain management, better medical care, and probably saves money.

An educational ethics program for surgical staff in the surgical intensive care unit (SICU) that addressed the issues of patient choice about dying, and the ethics of futile care, was associated with a decrease in length of stay from 28 to 16 days, and a decrease in SICU days from 2,028 to 1,003 days [57]. Again, the rapidly changing health care system could account for some of the change, but more ethically based care that valued the perspective of the patient [57] caused no increased costs.

Clinical practice guidelines for supportive care may decrease costs, but formal data have not been published (reviewed by Smith [52]). Standardization of care can improve the process of care even if not the outcomes. Clinical pathways for the surgical management of breast and lung cancer have improved short term results and lowered costs [58].

Table 6. Process or Structural Changes in care

Topic	Conclusion
Reducing uncontrolled pain admissions [56]	A system wide intervention of focus on pain management, a supportive care consultation team, and making a pain resource center. This was associated with a reduction in admissions from 255/5772 (4.4%) to 121/4076 (3.0%), at a projected cost savings of $2,719,245.
Coordinated nursing care manager for dying patients [54]	A nurse coordinator did not improve symptoms of dying patients, but did reduce overall costs by 41%, from £4774 to £8034. This was accomplished by a reduction in hospital days from 40 to 24, along with an increase in nurse home visits from 15 to 38. Patient and family satisfaction were not worsened.
Clinical practice guidelines for supportive care: anti-emetics, treatment of febrile neutropenia, treatment of pain [52,59,60]	A division changed practice to standardized oral anti-emetics, and once-daily ceftriaxone and gentamicin. Cost savings were estimated at $250,000 for each intervention, yearly.
Clinical practice pathways for care on lung and breast cancer patients undergoing diagnostic workup and surgery [58]	Pathways reduced variances in practice substantially, and generated cost savings. Care was thought to be improved.
Acquired immune deficiency care. First Boston Report, 1995 (unpublished data)	Up to a 50% reduction in total health care costs by reduced hospitalizations; home care visits increased by 600%. Financial details sketchy in this report, and data have not been published.
Presence of nursing care for end of life [55]	Nursing care availability allowed more patients to die at home consistent with the wishes of most patients.

Hospice vs. Non-Hospice Care

The available data cannot answer whether hospice improves care and saves money, or even improves care [52,61,62]. I have attempted to summarize the available data in Table 7.

A large randomized controlled trial of hospice vs. standard care is now 15 years old [63]. This study showed differences in medical outcomes or costs for patients randomized to hospice or standard care. The shortcomings of the study are several: 1) it was done at a Veterans Administration Medical Center and therefore included mostly male blue-collar workers, not representative of most hospice patients; 2) the hospice unit was newly formed and inexperienced and did not have routine referral lines (which probably would have precluded the study); and 3) the VAMC does not issue bills, so all costs were estimated using costs from nearby hospitals. The intervention was a special inpatient hospice unit with home care services for 247 patients in the trial, done in the period 1979-82. Hospice did not improve quality of care by any measured benchmark (pain, ability to perform activities of daily living). Patients still used many hospital days, 48 for control, 51 for hospice, but more of the hospice patients were hospitalized on the hospice unit. There was no difference in diagnostic procedures. Total costs of about $15,000 per patient showed no difference in the treatment groups. This study provides the best evidence that hospice will not have dramatic cost savings.

More recent data suggests that hospice care can be cost-saving, as long as the health care and payment systems are aligned with incentives to provide good care at the least acceptable cost as in Medicare [64]. In the 1992 Medicare files those who elected hospice were less costly than cancer patients who did not elect hospice. For those who enrolled in the last month of life, typically over half of Medicare patients, Medicare saved $1.65 for each $1 spent. Those who elected hospice tended to use more resources in the months from diagnosis until about three months before death, so the total disease management savings were much smaller (if any).

In an earlier similar analysis of 1988 data, Kidder found that Medicare hospice would save $1.26 for each $1 spent [65]. These savings were almost all from prevention of hospitalizations in the last month of life. Total disease management costs, or costs in the year preceding death, were similar in those who elected hospice and those who did not.

There is concern that hospice may actually not be saving total disease management costs, but just shifting them to costs not captured by our current accounting systems. In our own study of Medicare hospice use in Virginia, total disease management costs were actually higher for those who eventually elected hospice. Those who elect hospice tend to be high socioeconomic class patients with resources to absorb more home care costs, more out of pocket drug costs, etc. The data are consistent with an affluent group of patients using all the resources needed for treatment, then using hospice resources in addition. There is no data on whether the medically undeserved use hospice, will accept its philosophy, or how much those patients will cost the system. [52]

In a retrospective study of 12,000 patients at 40 centers, Aiken et al found that hospice patients were more likely to receive home nursing care, and spend less time in the hospital than conventional care patients [66]. These patients self-selected for hospice, so they may have used fewer or different resources anyway, and had more ability to absorb home care. Of the three models of care evaluated, conventional care was the least expensive when overall disease management costs were calculated, but hospital-based hospice ($2270) and home care hospice ($2657) were less expensive than conventional care ($6100) in the last month of life.

Table 7. Hospice vs. Non-Hospice Care

Topic	Conclusion
Randomized controlled trial of hospice vs. non-hospice care in Veterans Hospital [63]	Hospice did not improve or worsen quality of care by any measured benchmark (pain, ability to perform activities of daily living.). There was no difference in diagnostic procedures. Total costs were $15,000 per patient, with no difference in the arms.
Hospice election vs. Standard care, Medicare beneficiaries, 1992 [64]	Medicare saved $1.65 for each $1 spent on hospice programs; most of the savings occur during the last month of life
Hospice election vs. Standard care, Medicare beneficiaries, 1988 [65]	Medicare saved $1.26 for each $1 spent on hospice programs; most of the savings occur during the last month of life
Total costs from data bases [67]	No significant difference in total costs from diagnosis to death, but significant cost savings of 39% for hospice patients who were in hospice over two weeks.
Total disease management costs comparing those who elected hospice to those who did not [52]	No difference or slightly higher costs among Medicare beneficiaries who elected hospice. Within the hospice period, average 27 days, costs were slightly lower for those who elected hospice.
Home care [68,69]	Home care provided by relatives is not much different ($4,563 for each three month period) than costs in a nursing home or similar setting. The sicker the patient became, the more the cost to the family regardless of diagnosis. Costs were lowest when the patient and care giver lived in the same household.
Matching resource use to the dying patient [66]	Hospice patients more likely to receive more home nursing care, and spend less time in the hospital than conventional care patients. Conventional care was the least expensive when overall disease management costs were calculated, but hospital-based hospice ($2270) and home care hospice ($2657) were less expensive than conventional care ($6100) in the last month of life.

Use of Advanced Directives

In many countries, patients want to know their prognosis, and in the United States, physicians have ethical and legal obligations to inform them [70]. Advanced directives, such as "do not resuscitate" (DNR) orders, has been advocated to allow patients to make autonomous choices about their care at the end of life and possibly reduce costs by preventing futile care. However, as reviewed by Emanuel and Emanuel, there has been no cost savings associated either with the use of advanced directives or DNR orders. [61,71] (Table 8) These findings have been confirmed in the more recent SUPPORT study. [72]

Table 8. Use of Advanced Directives, Do Not Resuscitate Orders

Study	Conclusion
California Durable Power of Attorney for Health Care placed on chart [73]	No effect on treatment charges, types of treatment, or health status.
DNR [74]	Average of $57,334 for those without DNR orders, to $62,594 with those with DNR orders.
Advanced directives in SUPPORT hospitals [72]	No cost savings with advance directives. For patients prior to the SUPPORT intervention, there was a 23% reduction in cost associated with presence of advance directives, $21,284 with compared to $26,127 without. The intervention patients were more likely to have advance directives documented. Average cost was $24,178 for those without advanced directives, $28,017 for those with advanced directives on the intervention arm.

CONCLUSION

There are few good economic studies in palliative care. For some areas of care, such as coordination of care for the dying, the clinical benefit is not clear, but the cost-effectiveness evidence seems compelling enough to switch to coordinated care. Chemotherapy for some cancers (non-small cell lung cancer, prostate cancer, and gastrointestinal cancer) is reasonably effective and has acceptable cost-effectiveness ratios; this does not apply to any regimen that has not been formally evaluated. For other interventions, such as the use of advanced directives or hospice care, there is ethical and medical rationale, but little evidence so far that larger clinical benefit or cost savings will result.

REFERENCES

1. Brown ML: The national economic burden of cancer. *JNCI* 1990;82:1811-1814.

2. Brown ML, Hodgson TA, Rice DP: Economic impact of cancer in the U.S. in Schottenfeld D, Fraumeni J (eds): *Cancer, Epidemiology, and Prevention*. Oxford University Press; 1996:

3. Rundle RL: Salick Pioneers Selling Cancer Care to HMOs. *The Wall Street Journal* 1996;Monday, August 12:B1-B2.

4. Lubitz JD, Riley GF: Trends in Medicare payments in the last year of life. *N Engl J Med* 1993;328:1092-1096.

5. Lubitz J, Beebe J, Baker C: Longevity and Medicare expenditures. *N Engl J Med* 1995;332:999-1003.

6. Welch HG, Wennberg DE, Welch WP: The use of Medicare home health care services. *N Engl J Med* 1996;335:324-329.

7. Levinsky NG: The purpose of advance medical planning - autonomy for patients or limitation of care? *N Engl J Med* 1996;335:741-743.

8. Callahan D: Controlling the costs of health care for the elderly - fair means and foul. *N Engl J Med* 1996;335:744-746.

9. A controlled trial to improve care for seriously ill hospitalized patients. The study to understand prognoses and preferences for outcomes and risks of treatments (SUPPORT). The SUPPORT Principal Investigators. *JAMA* 1995;274:1591-1598.

10. Cleeland CS, Gonin R, Hatfield AK, et al: Pain and its treatment in outpatients with metastatic cancer. *N Engl J Med* 1994;330:592-596.

11. Farrow DC, Hunt WC, Samet JM: Geographic variation in the treatment of localized breast cancer. *N Engl J Med* 1992;326:1097-1101.

12. Nattinger AB, Gottlieb MS, Veum J, Yahnke D, Goodwin JS: Geographic variation in the use of breast-conserving treatment for breast cancer. *N Engl J Med* 1992;326:1102-1107.

13. Hillner BE, Penberthy L, Desch CE, McDonald K, Smith TJ, Retchin SR: Variation in staging and treatment of local and regional breast cancer in the elderly. *Breast Cancer Res Treatment* 1996;40:75-86.

14. Hillner BE, MacDonald MK, Penberthy L, et al: Measuring Standards of Care for Early Breast Cancer in an Insured Population. *Journal of Clinical Oncology* 1997;15:1401-1408.

15. Smith TJ, Penberthy L, Desch CE, et al: Differences in initial treatment patterns and outcomes of lung cancer in the elderly. *Lung Cancer* 1995;13:235-252.

16. Desch CE, Penberthy L, Newschaffer C, et al: Factors that Determine the Treatment of Local and Regional Prostate Cancer. *Med Care* 1996;34:152-162.

17. Gillis CR, Hole DJ: Survival outcome of care by specialist surgeons in breast cancer: a study of 3786 patients in the west of Scotland. *BMJ* 1996;312:145-148.

18. Sainsbury R, Haward R, Rider L, Johnstone C, Round C: Influence of clinician workload and patterns of treatment on survival from breast cancer. *Lancet* 1995;345:1265-1270.

19. Feuer EJ, Frey CM, Brawley OW, et al: After a treatment breakthrough: a comparison of trial and population-based data for advanced testicular cancer. *J Clin Oncol* 1994;12:368-377.

20. Nguyen HN, Averette HE, Hoskins W, Penalver M, Sevin B, Steren A: National survey of ovarian carcinoma Part V. The impact of physician's specialty on patient's survival. *Cancer* 1993;72:3663-3670.

21. Smith TJ, Desch CE, Hillner BE: Ways to reduce the cost of oncology care without compromising the quality. *Cancer Invest* 1994;12:257-265.

22. American Society of Clinical Oncology Outcomes Working Group (core members). Outcomes of cancer treatment for technology assessment and cancer treatment guidelines. *J Clin Oncol* 1995;14:671-679.

23. Slevin ML, Stubbs L, Plant HJ, et al: Attitudes to chemotherapy: comparing views of patients with cancer with those of doctors, nurses, and general public. *BMJ* 1990;300:1458-1460.

24. Davies E, Clarke C, Hopkins A: Malignant cerebral glioma - I: Survival, disability, and morbidity after radiotherapy. *BMJ* 1996;313:1507-1512.

25. Davies E, Clarke C, Hopkins A: Malignant cerebral glioma - II: Perspectives of patients and relatives on the value of radiotherapy. *BMJ* 1996;313:1512-1516.

26. Smith TJ, Hillner BE, Desch CE: Efficacy and cost-effectiveness of cancer treatment: rational allocation of resources based on decision analysis. *JNCI* 1993;85:1460-1474.

27. Laupacis A, Feeny D, Detsky AS, Tugwell PX: How attractive does a new technology have to be to warrant adoption and utilization? Tentative guidelines for using clinical and economic evaluation. *Can Med Assoc J* 1992;146:473-481.

28. Smith TJ: Which hat do I wear? *JAMA* 1993;270:1657-1659.

29. Blair SN, Kohl HW, III., Barlow CE, Paffenbarger RS, Jr., Gibbons LW, Macera CA: Changes in physical fitness and all-cause mortality. A prospective study of healthy and unhealthy men. *JAMA* 1995;273:1093-1098.

30. Souquet PJ, Chauvin F, Boissel JP, et al: Polychemotherapy in advanced non-small cell lung cancer: a meta-analysis. *Lancet* 1993;342:19-21.

31. Adelstein DJ: Palliative chemotherapy for non-small cell lung cancer. *Semin Oncol* 1995;22:35-39.

32. American Society of Clinical Oncology: Clinical Practice Guidelines for the Treatment of Unresectable Non-Small-Cell Lung Cancer. *Journal of Clinical Oncology* 1997;15:2996-3018.

33. Evans WK, Newman T, Graham I, et al: Lung Cancer Practice Guidelines: Lessons Learned and Issues Addressed by the Ontario Lung Cancer Disease Site Group. *Journal of Clinical Oncology* 1997;15:3049-3059.

34. Jaakimainen L, Goodwin PJ, Pater J, Warde P, Murray N, Rapp E: Counting the costs of chemotherapy in a National Cancer Institute of Canada randomized trial in non-small cell lung cancer. *J Clin Oncol* 1990;8:1301-1309.

35. Le Chevalier T, Brisgand D, Douillard JY, et al: Randomized study of vinorelbine and cisplatin versus vindesine and cisplatin versus vinorelbine alone in advanced non-small cell lung cancer: results of a European multicenter trial including 612 patients. *J Clin Oncol* 1994;12:360-367.

36. Smith TJ, Hillner BE, Neighbors DM, McSorley PA, Le Chevalier T: An economic evaluation of a randomized clinical trial comparing vinorelbine, vinorelbine plus cisplatin and vindesine plus cisplatin for non-small cell lung cancer. *J Clin Oncol* 1995;13:2166-2173.

37. Evans WK, Will BP, Berthelot JM, Earle CC: Cost of Combined Modality Interventions for Stage III Non-Small-Cell Lung Cancer. *Journal of Clinical Oncology* 1997;15:3038-3048.

38. Evans WK, Will BP: The cost of managing lung cancer in Canada. *Oncology Hunting* 1995;9:147-153.

39. Evans WK, Will BP, Berthelot JM, Wolfson MC: The economics of lung cancer management in Canada. *Lung Cancer* 1996;14:13-17.

40. Glimelius B, Hoffman K, Graf W, et al: Cost-effectiveness of palliative chemotherapy in advanced gastrointestinal cancer. *Ann Oncol* 1995;6:267-274.

41. Tannock IF, Osoba D, Stockler MR, et al: Chemotherapy With Mitoxantrone Plus Prednisone or Prednisone Alone for Symptomatic Hormone-Resistant Prostate Cancer: A Canadian Randomized Trial With Palliative End Points. *Journal of Clinical Oncology* 1996;14:1756-1764.

42. Bloomfield DJ, Krahn MD, Tannock IF, Smith TJ: Economic evaluation of chemotherapy with mitoxantrone plus prednisone for symptomatic hormone resistant prostate cancer (HRPC) based on a Canadian randomized trial (RCT) with palliative endpoints. *Proc Am Soc Clin Oncol* 1997;17:

43. Richards MA, Braysher S, Gregory WM, Rubens RD: Advanced breast cancer: use of resources and cost implications. *Br J Cancer* 1993;67:856-860.

44. Hillner BE, Smith TJ, Desch CE: Efficacy and cost-effectiveness of autologous bone marrow transplantation in metastatic breast cancer. Estimates using decision-analysis while awaiting clinical trial results. *JAMA* 1992;267:2055-2061.

45. Bezwoda WR, Seymour L, Dansey RD: High-dose chemotherapy with hematopoietic rescue as primary treatment for metastatic breast cancer: a randomized trial. *J Clin Oncol* 1995;13:2483-2489.

46. Welch HG, Larson EB: Cost-effectiveness of bone marrow transplantation in acute nonlymphocytic leukemia. *N Engl J Med* 1989;321:807-812.

47. Goodwin PJ, Feld R, Evans WK, Pater J: Cost-effectiveness of cancer chemotherapy: an economic evaluation of a randomized trial in small-cell lung cancer. *J Clin Oncol* 1988;6:1537-1547.

48. Ferris FD, Wodinsky HB, Kerr IG, Sone M, Hume S, Coons C: A cost-minimization study of cancer patients requiring a narcotic infusion in hospital and at home. *J Clin Epidemiol* 1991;44:313-327.

49. Wodinsky HB, DeAngelis C, Rusthoven JJ, et al: Re-evaluating the cost of outpatient cancer chemotherapy. *Can Med Assoc J* 1987;137:903-906.

50. Lowenthal RM, Piaszczyk A, Arthur GE, O'Malley S: Home chemotherapy for cancer patients: Cost analysis and safety. *Med J Aust* 1996;165:184-187.

51. Harris NJ, Dunmore R, Tscheu MJ: The Medicare hospice benefit: fiscal implications for hospice program management. *Cancer Management* 1996;May/June:6-11.

52. Smith TJ: End of Life Care: Preserving Quality and Quantity of Life in Managed Care. *ASCO Educ Book* 1997;33rd Annual Meeting:303-307.

53. Addington-Hall JM, MacDonald LD, Anderson HR, et al: Randomized controlled trial of effects of coordinating care for terminally ill cancer patients. *BMJ* 1992;305:1317-1322.

54. Raftery JP, Addington-Hall JM, MacDonald LD, et al: A randomized controlled trial of the cost-effectiveness of a district co-ordinating service for terminally ill cancer patients. *Palliat Med* 1996;10:151-161.

55. McWhinney IR, Bass MJ, Orr V: Factors associated with location of death (home or hospital) or patients referred to a palliative care team. *Can Med Assoc J* 1995;152:361-370.

56. Grant M, Ferrell BR, Rivera LM, Lee J: Unscheduled Readmissions for Uncontrolled Symptoms. *Nursing Clinics of North America* 1995;30:673-682.

57. Holloran SD, Starkey GW, Burke PA, Steele G, Jr., Forse RA: An educational intervention in the surgical intensive care unit to improve ethical decisions. *Surgery* 1995;118:294-298.

58. Katterhagen G: Physician compliance with outcome-based guidelines and clinical pathways in oncology. *Oncology* 1996;November:113-121.

59. Smith TJ: Reducing the cost of supportive care, Part I: Antibiotics for febrile neutropenia. *Clin Onc Alert* 1996;11:46-47.

60. Smith TJ: Reducing the cost of supportive care II: Anti-emetics. *Clin Onc Alert* 1996;11:62-64.

61. Emanuel EJ: Cost savings at the end of life. What do the data show? *JAMA* 1996;275:1907-1914.

62. Emanuel EJ, Emanuel LL: The economics of dying. The illusion of cost savings at the end of life. *N Engl J Med* 1994;330:540-544.

63. Kane RL, Berstein L, Whales J, Leibowitz A, Kaplan S: A randomized control trial of hospice care. *Lancet* 1984;1:890-894.

64. National Hospice Organization: *An analysis of the cost savings of the medicare hospice benefit*, Miami, FL, Lewin-VHI Inc; 1997:

65. Kidder D: The effects of hospice coverage on Medicare expenditures. *Health Serv Res* 1992;27:195-217.

66. Aiken LH: Evaluation and research and public policy: lessons learned from the National Hospice study. *J Chronic Dis* 1986;39:1-4.

67. Brooks CH, Smyth-Staruch K: Hospice home care cost savings to third party insurers. *Med Care* 1984;22:691-703.

68. Stommel M, Given CW, Given BA: The cost of cancer home care to families. *Cancer* 1993;71:1867-1874.

69. Given BA, Given CW, Stommel M: Family and out-of-pocket costs for women with breast cancer. *Cancer Pract* 1994;2:187-193.

70. Annas GJ: Informed consent, cancer, and truth in prognosis. *N Engl J Med* 1994;330:223-225.

71. Emanuel EJ, Emanuel LL: The Economics of Dying: The Illusion of Cost Savings at the End of Life. *The New England Journal of Medicine* 1994;330:540-544.

72. Teno J, Lynn J, Connors AF, Jr., et al: The illusion of end-of-life resource savings with advance directives. SUPPORT Investigators. Study to Understand Prognoses and Preferences for Outcomes and Risks of Treatment. *J Am Geriatr Soc* 1997;45:513-518.

73. Schneiderman LJ, Kronick R, Kaplan RM, Anderson JP, Langer RD: Effects of offering advance directives on medical treatments and costs. *Ann Intern Med* 1992;117:599-606.

74. Maksoud A, Jahnigen DW, Skibinski CI: Do not resuscitate orders and the cost of death. *Arch Intern Med* 1993;153:1249-1253.

ECONOMIC EVALUATION OF HEALTH CARE FOR CHRONIC DISEASES

Matthew H. Liang, MD, MPH

Department of Medicine, Division of Rheumatology, Immunology and Allergy, Harvard Medical School, Brigham and Women's Hospital, 75 Francis Street, Boston, MA 02115 USA

SUMMARY. The economic evaluation of health care services for chronic disease is an imperative borned of the fact that resources are finite; that technologic capacity and the public's demand for them have increased, and that choices are inevitable and difficult. Economic evaluation is an explicit and quantitative technique to provide qualitative assistance to those who must decide among competing uses of resources in situations of uncertainty. The forms of economic evaluation, cost of illness, cost minimization, cost-effectiveness, cost-benefit and cost-utility analyses are defined.

The economic evaluation paradigm has many methodological and conceptual problems for chronic disease. Until recently no methodological standards existed. Even with these the identification and assessment of costs, the measurement of health benefits and the valuation of health benefits - key elements - remain unstandardized. Valuation research attempts to quantitate the utilities of health states but some groups (the elderly, the uneducated, minorities) cannot deal with the questions posted and implies that their perceptions are selectively excluded from studies that will inform health policy. Chronic rheumatic disease are lifelong. All areas of function can be affected and the types of interventions, medical surgical, rehabilitation, psychosocial, vocational, are varied in their application over time and in intensity. Economic studies are short term and focused on single interventions- all inappropriate for chronic disease. In the final analysis, like it or not, the question of what health care is worth societal investment is debated in every organized system of health care delivery. This should not be done nor interpreted by only a part of the stakeholders, nor without empirical data and the input of providers, patients and potential patients.

KEY WORDS: Cost-benefit, Cost-effectiveness, Cost-minimization, Chronic disease

INTRODUCTION

The economic evaluation of health care in general and for chronic diseases has become imperative in modern societies. It is borned from the fact that resources are finite, that the technologic capacity and the public's demand for health care have increased. The choices for the use of resources had become more explicit, inevitable and difficult. In the United States, dissemination of palliative care for terminal patients has been limited by funding allowed or available for the nursing personnel and the facilities to house patients for their terminal course(1).

The objective of economic evaluation is to assist decision makers in choosing among competing alternatives in situations of uncertainty and limited resources by providing quantitative analysis for qualitative insight(2,3). Underlying its application are the assumptions that choices are inevitable and that implicit value judgments can be made more explicit and that all decisions involve balancing costs and benefits. Economic evaluation, however, is not about indiscriminate cost-cutting, about identifying the cheapest and most effective or necessarily the "right answer". Most importantly they should not be applied to patient care decisions. With this preamble, this paper describes the major types of economic evaluation used in health care and discusses its limitations for decision making in chronic disease management.

DEFINITION OF TERMS

A formal economic evaluation involves a comparison of the costs and health effects of the clinically relevant alternatives. The analysis of the costs is equivalent for all types of economic evaluation and the types of economic evaluation only differ in the way health effects are measured. Direct medical costs include costs of medical treatment such as professional services, tests, medication, hospitalizations and home care services. Direct non-medical costs include transportation to and from a health care facility, home and work-site modifications to adapt an environment for better function, and other costs attributable to the medical condition. Direct costs are differentiated from charges which are billed to the patient in some health care systems. These include overhead and other costs which can be idiosyncratic to the organization.

Indirect costs are work gains or lost income due to the medical condition measured by the difference between expected and actual earnings. In comparing different approaches or techniques, the most relevant ratio is the incremental cost-effectiveness and not the average cost-effectiveness. The incremental cost-effectiveness ratio answers the question of whether the difference in costs divided by the difference in effectiveness between two alternative strategies justifies the use of more effective strategy.

Economic analyses of medical and surgical care have gained a firm foothold in the medical literature but many physicians have had little background to independently judge their quality and few standards have been articulated until recently. Some questions of the article to keep in mind are outlined in Table 1; for more detailed discussion, the interested reader is referred to recent publications on this subject (4,5,6).

TYPES OF ECONOMIC EVALUATIONS

Cost of Illness Study

Cost of illness studies which look only at the cost side or cost impact are not economic evaluations in a strict sense. They may provide, however, important information on the cost of a health program.

The costs of chronic illnesses are usually higher than those of acute illnesses because the costs over the lifetime, albeit occasionally shortened, of individual.

Cost studies provide data on costs in different settings and serve as a basis to measure efficiency. However, if one wants to compare the costs in different settings meaningfully, controlling for characteristics related to outcome such as age, comorbid illness is essential.

Cost Analysis

Any economic evaluation that compares at least two alternative strategies is a cost analysis. If both alternatives have similar risk-benefit ratios an evaluation might focus only on the cost side of the equation.

To society the costs of a health care intervention are the costs from consuming resources minus the cost savings which are returns to the resource pool. Methodological issues common to all cost-analyses are questions of how to obtain cost data, how to discount future costs and whether the study question is posed in terms of society, the individual, the payer or the clinician. Although obtaining actual costs is the most rigorous way to get the data, practically one is often restricted to the use of charges or estimates of average costs for specific interventions or services. Costs occurring in the future are generally discounted to its present value (typically with a discount rate of 5%, a rate which is similar to the long-term interest rate (2). Depending on one's perspective, direct and indirect costs may be either expenditures or savings. For example, hospital costs are often not a cost to the patient but to the health insurance and the society.

Cost-analyses comparing different treatments for a given chronic illness implicitly assume equivalent risk-effectiveness ratios for the treatment alternatives which is not correct; e.g.. in the comparison of revision and resection arthroplasty the effectiveness of revision surgery is better but has a higher complication rate.

Cost-Minimization Analysis

In cost-minimization evaluations the question is asked, "What is the least costly alternative?" and the focus is only on comparison of costs. Implicit or undealt with are that the health outcomes are equivalent. There is no attempt to balance costs against benefits. In chronic diseases whether or not health care services are provided may not be an issue but how the care can be provided more economically is and cost minimization strategies can be fruitful

Cost-Benefit Analysis

In cost-benefit analysis (CBA) health effects are valued in monetary terms (johannesson90[12]). A CBA calculates the difference of costs and health effects. An intervention should be performed if it increases the total utility for society, which is the case when the monetary value of the health effects exceed the costs. In comparing alternative strategies, the program resulting in the largest difference is preferred. The main and unresolved problem with DBA is the validity of measuring the monetary value of health effects. The most common method uses expressed preference in the format of the maximal willingness to pay (7).

Cost-Effectiveness Analysis

A cost effectiveness analysis (CEA) compares the costs of an intervention to the main effect. From the intervention the main effect is typically measured in physical units such as blood pressure, bone density, units of pain or physical function. One limitation with this approach is that only one outcome is included in the equation. Other health effects and, importantly, adverse effects are typically not included in the analysis. However, the use of a global health status instrument which integrates pain and physical, psychological and social function addresses all relevant outcome dimensions for the evaluation of treatment in chronic disease management. CEA does not allow comparison with other health care programs unless the endpoints studied are the same across these programs.

CEA may be considered a useful first step in exploring the magnitude of the incremental cost-effectiveness of different strategies for chronic disease. To study chronic disease management, it would be ideal to use a general health status instrument that measures pain and physical function, the main goals of chronic disease management.

Cost-Utility Analysis

In cost-utility analysis (CUA) (8) a common measure of outcome is used. "Utility" is the value of a particular health state and is measured in 'quality adjusted life years' (QALYs: life expectancy weighted for quality of life (8). Although the estimation of QALYs has problems, particularly the elicitation of individual preferences, it's useful to compare different health care interventions because it integrates different health effects and side effects and uses a common measure of outcome.

By identifying which figures influence or "drive" the results one can also identify the critical costs or probabilities which could be modified to improve the cost-utility of an intervention.

Direct medical costs are usually the most important costs influencing the cost-utility ratio.

The impact of **indirect costs** has had limited study. Indirect costs due to maintained or regained work capacity may be of less importance than in interventions for patients close to the age of retirement. However, in young and active patients with congenital or traumatic causes of chronic diseases, earlier treatment and consequently earlier complications of treatment may occur.

Savings of indirect costs from reduced use of social services and nursing home placement may be influential to the cost-utility of health interventions for elderly patients. Support from significant others, continence and intact cognitive function may be more important than functional capacity. In patients with multiple medical problems, the improved function from any intervention for one of these problems may not affect independence.

Increased **operative morbidity and mortality** are critical and influential variables in populations with complicated medical and surgical histories who undergo a surgical intervention. Any treatment with reduced morbidity and mortality would be evaluated to advantage in such situations. Future health benefits are less important in the cost-utility ratio of a more effective treatment because of a decreased life-expectancy and therefore smaller future cumulative health gains.

STRENGTHS AND LIMITATIONS OF THE ECONOMIC EVALUATION PARADIGM

Consideration of 'who should get what' and 'who shall suffer' raise ethical questions and collide with the traditional role of the physician as the advocate of his patients irrespective of costs. Unfortunately, clinical practice without consideration of costs endangers other useful social and health care programs. Performed carefully with valid data (and interpreted cautiously) economic analyses can make difficult judgments more explicit and rational. Physicians should understand rather than fear them.

For chronic diseases, the economic evaluation paradigm presents special conceptual, methodological, and ethical problems (9). Until very recently (7) although the steps by which such analyses were done were similar, the details of the methods were not standardized. For instance the basic preference measurement or weight of health benefits have not been standardized and the techniques for their measurement not examined for their comprehension, validity, reliability or response bias. In our own work we have found willingness-to-pay is a concept which defies many elderly; and in those who can understand the question, the response is heavily driven by the persons income. The time-trade-off method tends to be less sensitive in less educated and in younger patients (10). Health policy should strive for fairness and equity and using measures that only some can answer or understand presents major concerns.

Chronic disease management is driven by the multiple changing needs of a patient over time. As a consequence its management frequently involves multiple disciplines which have to be coordinated and adjusted repeatedly. Even seemingly simple interventions such as joint arthroplasty involves a complex number of discrete medical, surgical, rehabilitation, nursing cointerventions to achieve the best results. Economic evaluation by necessity simplifies multiple complex interventions where the contribution of the components can not easily be deconstructed and it's important that clinicians resist the attempts of analysis to fragment comprehensive multidisciplinary interventions into its component parts.

Chronic diseases, by definition, do not significantly shorten life. Economic evaluations must factor into estimates the host of complexities that occur over the life of an individual such as the accumulation of concomitant medical/surgical problems; the slow downward trajectory of functional ability; and the availability of a social support system or care takers which is the critical determinant, often, of institutionalization. These are important factors which are difficult to model and to measure.

Finally, posing the problem of allocating health resources as an economic one changes a discussion from one of defining social values to one of dollars and cents. In the process, the real question and the real answers are obscured by "hard" numbers.

For all its limitations, choice is difficult and economic evaluations should be viewed as decision aids, not the truth. Physicians should understand their assumptions so that they can be properly interpreted.

Acknowledgments

I'm grateful to Dr. Hideki Hashimoto who provided invaluable comments and Ms Rita DeLuca who cheerfully and professionally produced this paper.

REFERENCES

1. Meier DE, Morrison RS, Cassel CK (1997) Improving Palliative Care. Ann Int Med; 127:225-230.

2. Weinstein MC (1990) Principles of cost-effective resource allocation in health care organizations. Int J Techn Assessm Health Care 6:93-103.

3. Johannesson M, Jonsson B (1991) Economic evaluation in health care: is there a role for cost-benefit analysis? Health Policy 17:1-23.

4. Drummond MF, Richardson WS, O'Brien BJ, Levine M, Heyland D (1997) Users' Guides to the Medical Literature XIII. How to Use an Article on Economic Analysis of Clinical Practice. Are the Results Valid. JAMA 277:1552-1557.

5. Russell LB et al (1996) The Role of Cost-Effectiveness Analysis in Health Medicine. JAMA 276;1172-1177.

6. Kassirer JP, Angell M (1994) The Journal's Policy on Cost-Effectiveness Analysis. NEJM 331:669-670.

7. Weinstein MC et al (1996) Recommendations of the Panel on Cost-Effectiveness in Health and Medicine. JAMA 276:1253-1258.

8. Torrance GW. Measurement of health state utilities for economic appraisal. A review. J Health Economics 1986;5:1-30.

9. Wynig MK (1997) Economic Analyses, the Medical Commons and Patients' Dilemmas: What is the Physician's Role? J Investigative Medicine 45: 35-43.

10. Katz JN, Phillips CB, Fossel AH, Liang MH. Stability and responsiveness of utility measures. Med Care 1994;32:183-188.

RECENT TREND AND PROBLEMS OF HEALTH ECONOMICS IN JAPAN: APPLICATION OF CLINICAL ECONOMICS TO THE TREATMENT FOR CANCERS AND INTRACTABLE DISEASES

Akinori Hisashige

Department of Preventive Medicine, University of Tokushima, School of Medicine, 3-18-15 Kuramoto, Tokushima, 770 Japan

SUMMARY. While Japan's healthcare system has achieved accessibility and equity of healthcare, the most serious problem it faces is unassured quality and efficiency of healthcare. To promote reforms of the healthcare system, the Japanese government emphasized the urgent need for the establishment of economic evaluation of healthcare. Responding to this situation, in the area of treatment of cancers and intractable diseases, economic evaluation has been carried out. Several examples of economic evaluations, such as bone marrow transplantation for leukemias, breast conserving treatment for early breast cancer, and antiemetic treatment for patients receiving cancer chemotherapy, showed substantial possibilities for evaluating value for money of healthcare to establish an effective and efficient healthcare system.

KEY WORDS: Health economics, Decision analysis, Cancer treatment, Liver transplantation, Bone marrow transplantation

INTRODUCTION

Faced with an explosion in healthcare costs, aging population and healthcare technology growth, coupled with a decline in economic growth, developed countries have directed attention to evidence-based health care combined with health economics to maximize health benefits at low costs [1-3]. As is shown in Figure 1, the number of publications mentioning economic aspects of health care has been increasing, in particular since 1990.

While Japan's healthcare system has achieved accessibility and equity of healthcare, the

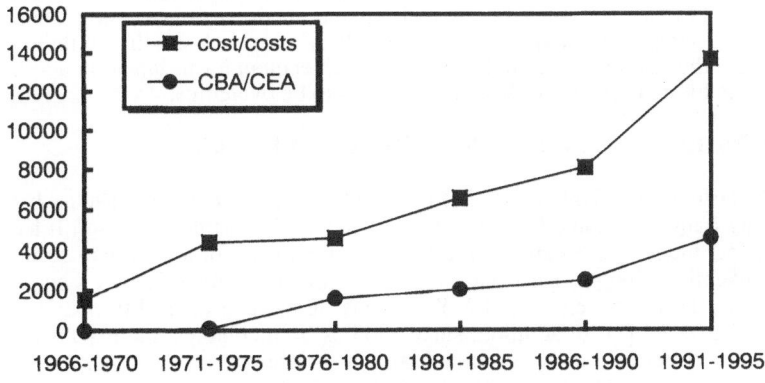

Figure 1 Number of publications mentioning economic aspects classified by years (MEDLINE: 1966-1995). Abbreviations: CBA=cost-benefit analysis; CEA=cost-effectiveness analysis.

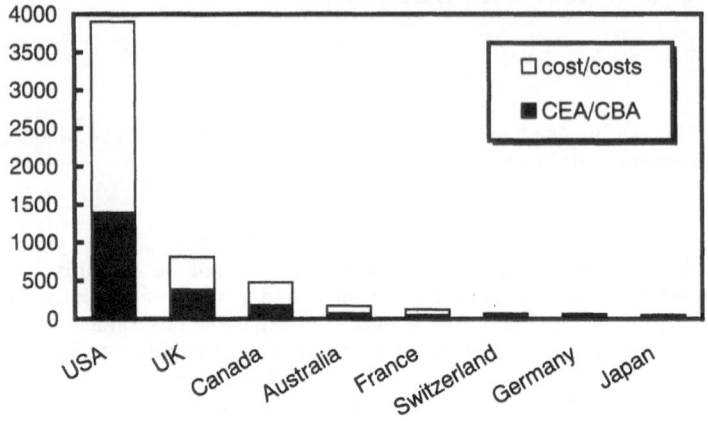

Number of publications

Figure 2   Number of publications mentioning economic aspects
classified by country of origin (MEDLINE:1986-1995).
CBA and CEA are the same as in Figure 1.

most serious problem it faces is unassured quality and efficiency of healthcare. In particular, the Japanese government has no explicit health policy to comprehensively evaluate effectiveness and efficiency of healthcare [1]. Under these circumstances, activities of economic evaluations for healthcare in Japan have been very limited compared with those in other developed countries (Figure 2).

However, in recent years, a drastic change has been observed. To promote reforms of healthcare system, the Japanese government emphasized the urgent need for establishment of economic evaluation, in particular for drugs, as well as healthcare technology assessment [1]. This action has had a dramatic effect on economic evaluation of healthcare among pharmaceutical industries and healthcare professionals.

Responding to this situation, in the area of treatment of cancers and intractable diseases, economic evaluation has been introduced. For example, we have carried out several economic evaluations in this area such as bone marrow transplantation for leukemias, breast conserving treatment for early breast cancer, antiemetic treatment for patients receiving cancer chemotherapy, liver transplantation for biliary atresia. According to these evaluations, we examined the possibility of application of health economics in Japan. In addition, we also identified the future problems of health economics to be overcome.

1. BONE MARROW TRANSPLANTATION FOR LEUKEMIAS

Bone marrow transplantation (BMT) was introduced in the early 1960s. It has become increasingly frequent among developed countries over the last decade [4-6]. It has developed from an experimental procedure to an established treatment for a variety of serious disorders such as leukemias, Hodgkin's disease, aplastic anemia, immunodeficiency syndromes, and so on. However, the effectiveness of BMT in terms of survival or quality of life has not been fully established yet [7]. In addition, since BMT is both complex and expensive technology requiring extensive and costly coordination, it is considered to be one of the factors in the escalation of health care costs [6-8]. To identify problems in introducing BMT into Japan, economic evaluation for BMT was carried out.

As is shown in Table 1, to evaluate the efficiency of BMT in Japan, a retrospective cohort study and cost-effectiveness analysis [9] of BMT for acute leukemia (AL) and chronic myeloid leukemia (CML) were carried out. In economic evaluation, a payer's viewpoint [9] was adopted for the estimation of costs. Only direct costs were evaluated. The observation period of the cohort study was 5 years. Under the condition extrapolated beyond 5 years, each survivor was assigned a life expectancy equal to the Japanese average. As a comparator of BMT, chemotherapy was used. In addition, no treatment strategy, where patients would die rapidly, was also considered. Life years gained was used as an index of health outcome for each strategy.

The subjects were patients admitted to a public hospital in Osaka during 1983 and 1987. The number of patients for BMT and chemotherapy for acute leukemia (AL) was 12 and 11, respectively. The average age among them was 20.5 and 25.5, respectively. In the case of chronic myeloid leukemia (CML), the number of patients for BMT and chemotherapy was 12 and 26, respectively. The average age here was 24.4 and 33.3.

As regards BMT, among AL cases, patients who achieved 1st complete remission were offered it. For CML, patients during the chronic phase were offered it. Before receiving it, conditioning (high dose of cyclophoshamide and total body irradiation) was undergone, and short-term methotrexate and cyclosporine were given for prevention of graft versus host disease. On the other hand, in the case of chemotherapy for AL, the protocol [10] according to the Japan Adult Leukemia Study Group was used. Since interferon-alpha for CML was not introduced until the 1990s in Japan [11], only conventional chemotherapy such as hydroxy urea etc was administered to these subjects.

Table 2 shows the costs and health outcome per patient of BMT and chemotherapy. The costs during the 5 year period for BMT and chemotherapy were $180,400 and $136,500, respectively. Life years gained in comparison with no treatment from BMT and chemotherapy were 4.24 and 2.96. In the case of lifetime follow up, costs in both alternatives were $180,700 and $180,700. Life years gained were 39.04 and 19.10. At five year follow up, the cost-effectiveness (CE) ratios of BMT and chemotherapy for AL were $45,000 and $48,000 per life year gained, respectively (Table 3). Incremental CE ratio of BMT over chemotherapy was $33,300 per life year gained. On the other hand, at lifetime follow up, CE ratios for BMT and chemotherapy were $12,600 and $19,500, respectively. Incremental CE ratio was $4,600. The two-way sensitivity analysis of incremental CE ratio according to discount rate for effectiveness and costs showed that it varied from $33,000 to $41,300.

Table 1   Cost-effectiveness analysis of BMT for acute leukemia and chronic myeloid leukemia

Object: To compare efficiency of BMT for acute leukemia and chronic myeloid leukemia with chemotherapy (and do nothing)	
Study design	: CEA, Retrospective analysis
Standpoint	: Payer
Effectiveness	: Retrospective cohort study
Comparator	: Chemotherapy, do nothing
Outcome	: Life years gained
Costs	: Direct costs
Study period	: 5 years, lifetime
Efficiency	: Cost-effectiveness ratio ($/life year gained)
Discount rate	: 5% (costs and effectiveness)

Table 2   Costs and health outcomes of BMT and chemotherapy for acute leukemia

Therapy	Costs($)		Life years gained	
	5 year	lifetime	5 year	lifetime
Chemotherapy	136,500	180,700	2.96	19.10
BMT	180,400	180,700	4.24	39.04

Exchange rate is 100 yen = US$1

Table 4 shows the costs and health outcome per patient of BMT and chemotherapy. The costs during the 5 year period for BMT and chemotherapy were $132,900 and $52,000, respectively. Life years gained in comparison with no treatment from BMT and chemotherapy were 4.34 and 3.04. In case of lifetime follow-up, costs in both alternatives were $133,500 and $68,500. Life years gained were 38.40 and 8.79. At 5 year follow-up, the cost-effectiveness (CE) ratios of BMT and chemotherapy for CML were $32,200 and $16,600 per life year gained, respectively (Table 5). Incremental CE ratio of BMT over chemotherapy was $72,200 per life year gained. On the other hand, at lifetime follow-up, CE ratios of BMT and chemotherapy were $9,200 and $11,500, respectively. Incremental CE ratio was $8,100. The two-way sensitivity analysis of incremental CE ratio according to discount rate for effectiveness and costs showed that it varied from $61,800 to $77,300.

These results show that BMT for AL is likely to be more efficient than chemotherapy at the five year follow up. Moreover, since life years gained in BMT are longer than those in chemotherapy, incremental analysis [9] shows that change of strategy from chemotherapy to BMT is also efficient. Sensitivity analysis confirmed these results. In addition, if costs and effectiveness are projected to lifetime, the efficiency of BMT is estimated to be increasing very rapidly. On the other hand, although BMT and chemotherapy were indicated to be more efficient for CML than they were for AL, BMT was less efficient than chemotherapy in CML at 5 years follow-up. However, life years gained in BMT are longer than in chemotherapy. Incremental efficiency of BMT over chemotherapy in CML is $72,200 which is slightly higher than that in AL. In lifetime follow-up, BMT is suspected to be more efficient than chemotherapy even in CML. Incremental CE ratio in CML is the same as that in AL.

Table 3   Cost-effectiveness ratio of BMT for acute leukemia (5 year follow-up)

Therapy	Cost-effectiveness ratio ($ per life year gained)
Chemotherapy	48,000
BMT	45,000
Chemotherapy → BMT	33,300

(Discount: 5% for costs and effectiveness)

Table 4   Costs and health outcomes of BMT and chemotherapy for chronic myeloid leukemia

Therapy	Costs ($)		Life years gained	
	5 years	lifetime	5 years	lifetime
Chemotherapy	52,000	68,500	3.04	8.79
BMT	132,900	133,500	4.34	38.40

Table 5   Cost-effectiveness ratio of BMT for chronic myeloid leukemia (5 year follow-up)

Therapy	Cost-effectiveness ratio ($ per life year gained)
Chemotherapy	16,600
BMT	32,200
Chemotherapy → BMT	72,200

(Discount: 5% for both costs and outcomes)

Although there are several differences in methods, costs and health outcomes, the results in this study are consistent with those [6,8] reported before in the U.S.

In Japan, the introduction and utilization of BMT were not linked to any formal assessment in health policy. In this study, considerable potentiality for efficacy and efficiency of BMT was observed. For the future, the effectiveness and efficiency of BMT need to be comprehensibly evaluated for appropriate and efficient utilization of BMT.

2. BREAST CONSERVING TREATMENT FOR EARLY BREAST CANCER

In the late 1980s, randomized controlled trials have shown that there is no statistical difference in survival between breast conserving treatment (BCT) and mastectomy for early breast cancer [12,13]. Since BCT is less invasive than mastectomy, it is an important option for treatment of early breast cancer. Benefits and risks including quality of life with BCT have been extensively examined in the US and European countries [14-17]. BCT has been indicated as the first choice for treatment of early breast cancer by a consensus development conference [13]. In contrast, in Japan, no systematic evaluation of BCT has been carried out. Its diffusion still remains at a quite low level. While this situation will damage patients' quality of life, it should be evaluated from the perspectives of both clinical practice and health policy. Evaluation of effectiveness and efficiency of BCT for early breast cancer in Japan was carried out (Table 6).

To evaluate the prognosis and complications of BCT and its competitive alternative, mastectomy, in Japan, a critical evaluation and meta-analysis [18] of existing information, which was identified through the computer search for information mentioned above, was carried out. Quality of life (utility) [9] of health outcomes after treatment for breast cancer was evaluated. A time-trade off method [9] was used for utility measurement. The subjects were 98 medical and nursing students. Finally, to evaluate efficacy and efficiency of BCT in Japan, a cost-effectiveness analysis and cost-utility analysis of BCT for early breast cancer were carried out using a Markov model [19] (Figure 3). In economic evaluation, a payer's viewpoint was adopted for the estimation of costs. Only direct costs were evaluated. The endpoint of the observation period was set at the age of 80. As a comparator of BCT, mastectomy was used. Life years gained and quality adjusted life years (QALYs) [9] were used as an index of health outcome for each strategy.

In Japan, evidence of effectiveness of BCT was based on a case study with a relatively large number of subjects and several retrospective historical cohort studies [20]. The results of meta-analysis of this information is shown in Table 7. While the survival rate and those after local recurrence and distant metastasis were higher in BCT than in mastectomy, local recurrence and distant metastasis rates were also higher in BCT. Utility of health states after

Table 6 Cost-effectiveness and cost-utility analysis of breast conserving treatment for early breast cancer

Object: To evaluate effectiveness and efficiency of breast conserving treatment in comparison with mastectomy	
Study design	: CEA, CUA, Retrospective analysis
Standpoint	: Payer
Effectiveness	: Meta analysis of published papers, Markov model
Comparator	: Mastectomy
Outcome	: Life years gained (LY), Quality adjusted life years (QALY)
Costs	: Direct costs
Study period	: Lifetime
Efficiency	: Cost-effectiveness ratio ($/LY), Cost-utility ratio ($/QALY)
Discount rate	: 5% (costs and outcomes)

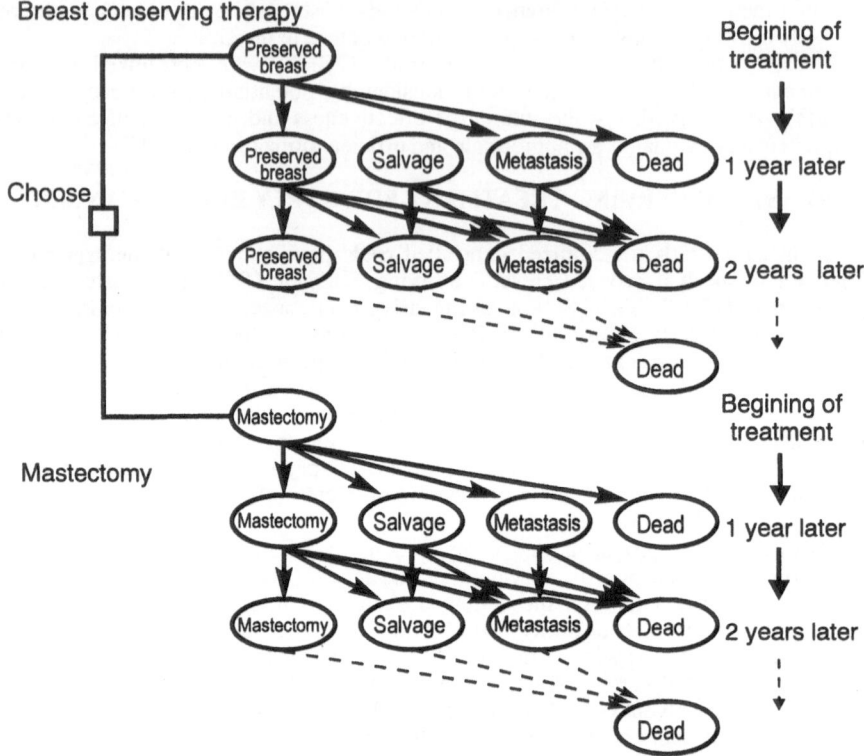

Figure 3 Decision analysis for treatment of early
breast cancer by a Markov model

Table 7 Health outcomes for therapy of early breast cancer
estimated by meta-analysis (during a period of 5 years follow up)

	%
Breast conserving therapy	
survival rate	97.79
local recurrence rate	6.79
distant metastasis rate	4.38
survival rate after local recurrence	76.00
survival rate after distant metastasis	25.35
Mastectomy	%
survival rate	96.84
local recurrence rate	2.46
distant metastasis rate	2.82
survival rate after local recurrence	53.00
survival rate after distant metastasis	13.33

BCT and mastectomy is shown in Table 8. Utility value (0.86) for preserved breast was slightly higher than that (0.80) for mastectomy. That of health state after salvage surgery and metastasis were 0.67 and 0.40, respectively. These results are consistent with the results of utility measurement in other countries [21].

As is shown in Table 9, expected life years (LYs) and quality adjusted life years (QALYs) after BCT at 40 years old were 32.98 and 27.66, respectively. Both LYs and QALYs in BCT were higher than those in mastectomy. These results were consistent with those at 50 and 60 years old. Table 10 shows results of economic evaluation of BCT. Incremental cost-effectiveness (CE) ratio and cost-utility (CU) ratio of BCT compared with mastectomy at 40 years old were 9,490 ($/LY) and 3,220 ($/QALY), respectively. Sensitivity analysis of incremental CE and CU ratios according to age showed that they varied from 9,490 to 23,420, and from 3,220 to 3,730, respectively. In addition, sensitivity analysis according to discount rate (3%, 5%, 7%) showed that incremental CE and CU ratios varied from 7,130 to 10,720, and from 2,870 to 3,340, respectively.

Table 8　Quality of life (utility) of breast cancer

Health outcomes	Utility values
Healthy	1.00
preserved breast	0.86
mastectomy	0.80
salvage	0.67
metastasis	0.40
Dead	0.00

Numerical value (Median): time trade-off

Table 9　Decision analysis of prognosis for treatment of early breast cancer (stressed on radiation therapy after breast conserving treatment).

Health outcomes	BCT		MT
40 years old			
expected life years	32.98	>	32.07
expected QALYs	27.66	>	25.39
50 years old			
expected life years	25.33	>	24.62
expected QALYs	21.22	>	19.46
60 years old			
expected life years	17.40	>	17.03
expected QALYs	14.62	>	13.45

QALYs (Quality Adjusted Life Years)

Table 10　Incremental cost-effectiveness ratio and cost-utility ratio of breast conserving therapy (40 years old)

Measures	Estimation
Cost-effectiveness ratio	9,490　($/LY)
Cost-utility ratio	3,220 ($/QALY)

Discount rate: 5% both cost and outcome
LY: life years gained
QALY: Quality adjusted life years gained

These results show that BCT for early breast cancer is likely to be more efficient than mastectomy, in particular when quality of life is taken into consideration. While sensitivity analysis confirmed these results, BCT was more efficient at younger age. Although there are several differences in subjects, methods, health outcomes, and quality of life measurement, the results for prognosis after BCT or mastectomy in this study are consistent with those reported before based on data from other countries [21]. Cost-effectiveness and cost-utility analysis showed that BCT is efficient treatment in comparison with mastectomy. Based on these results, health policy and clinical guidelines for appropriate and efficient adoption and utilization of BCT should be realized.

3. ANTIEMETIC TREATMENT FOR PATIENTS RECEIVING CANCER CHEMOTHERAPY

Nausea and emesis are common adverse effects of chemotherapy for cancer and are primary concerns of patients receiving chemotherapy [22]. The concerns of these adverse effects can be classified in several ways such as patients' quality of life, costs of cancer therapy, patients' time lost for work, and so on [23]. The advent of a new class of antiemetic drugs, antagonists to the serotonin receptor subtype 5-HT3 has significantly reduce the incidence of nausea and emesis [24]. However, the relative high cost of these new drugs has generated debate about their use [25]. To address this issue, economic evaluation of a new 5-HT3 receptor antagonist (tropisetron) was carried out.

As is shown in Table 11, to evaluate the efficiency of antiemetic treatment, a retrospective cost-minimization analysis [9] and cost-effectiveness analysis [9] based on randomized controlled trials were done. As a comparator, placebo with conventional care for nausea and emesis was used. A payer's viewpoint was adopted for the estimation of costs, and only direct costs were evaluated. However, since no difference was observed in the period of hospitalization between alternatives, a payer's viewpoint is similar to a societal viewpoint. Incidence of emesis or significant emesis (more than two episodes) in the first 24 hours was used as an index of health outcome for each strategy.

Table 12 shows the cost of dealing with emesis per episode. The cost of care by a nurse was \$3.16, and its main component was costs of nursing time. On the other hand, the cost of treatment was \$65.05, and its main components were costs of physicians and antiemetic regimen. The result of cost-minimization analysis showed that total costs of antiemetic treatment by tropisetron and placebo per patient were \$45.3 and \$107.0, respectively (Table 13). Although antiemetic treatment increased costs due to antiemetic drug, it decreased further costs for dealing with emesis. Moreover, the costs and effectiveness of antiemetic treatment by tropisetron are shown in Table 14. Reduction of incidence of emesis and significant emesis per patient were 31.5% and 57.0%, respectively. The costs of antiemetic

Table 11 Cost-minimization and cost-effectiveness analysis of antiemetic treatment by tropisetron

Object: To evaluate efficiency of antiemetic treatment by 5-HT3 receptor antagonist for patients receiving cancer chemotherapy	
Study design	: CMA, CEA, Retrospective analysis
Standpoint	: Payer
Effectiveness	: Randomized controlled trials
Comparator	: Placebo
Outcome	: Incidence of emesis
Costs	: Direct costs
Study period	: 24 hours
Efficiency	: Cost-effectiveness ratio (\$/episode of emesis prevented)

Table 12 Costs of dealing with emesis per episode

Item	Costs ($)
Care for emesis	
Nursing time (8.8 min)	2.42
Linen, disposals	0.75
Subtotal	3.16
Treatment for emesis	
Doctor's time (14.2 min)	10.76
Nursing time (6.3 min)	1.73
Drugs	50.37
Disposals	2.18
Subtotal	65.05

Table 13 Costs of antiemetic treatment (per patient)

Items	Tropisetron	Placebo
Costs of antiemetic drugs	$22.17	-
Costs dealting with emetics	$23.13	$106.99
Total	$45.30	$106.99

Table 14 Cost and effectiveness of antiemetic treatment by tropisetron in comparison with placebo

Items	Significant emesis	Emesis
Emesis prevented	57.0%	31.5%
Costs	-$61.69	-$61.69
Cost-effectiveness ratio	-$108.23	-$195.84

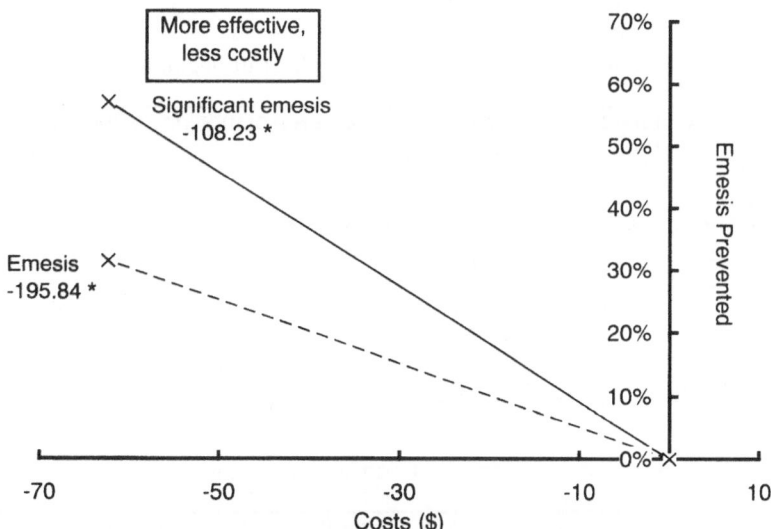

Figure 4 Cost-effectiveness of antiemetic treatment by tropisetron (in comparison with placebo).
* average cost-effectiveness ratio ($).

treatment for emesis and significant emesis per patient were -$61.7. The cost effectiveness ratios were -$195.8 and -$108.2 per episode prevented for emesis and significant emesis (Table 14 and Figure 4).

These results show that antiemetic treatment by tropisetron was not only effective but also cost saving in comparison with placebo.

4. LIVER TRANSPLANTATION FOR BILIARY ATRESIA

Organ transplantations are provided all over the world for patients with end-stage heart, liver or renal failure [26,27]. Although there is no formal experimental evaluation of its effectiveness, analysis of case series showed more and more favourable results. Organ transplantations are no longer considered experimental. However, organ transplantation is expensive high medical technology which has the potential for the escalation of health care expenditure [26,27]. To examine cost-effectiveness of organ transplantation in Japan, economic evaluation was carried out. As a typical example of organ transplantation in Japan, living liver transplantation for infants with biliary atresia was selected. Biliary atresia is idiopathic, inflammatory obstruction of extrahepatic bile ducts among infants. It accounts for the single most frequent cause of death due to liver disease in infancy and childhood in Japan.

Table 15 shows a study design to evaluate the efficiency of liver transplantation (LT). A retrospective cohort study and cost-effectiveness analysis [9] based on it were carried out. In economic evaluation, a payer's viewpoint was adopted for the estimation of costs. Only direct costs were evaluated. The observation period of the cohort study based on registry data on LT was 6 years. Under the condition extrapolated beyond 6 years, each survivor was assigned a life expectancy equal to the Japanese average. As a comparator of LT, hepatic portoenterostomy (HP) [28] which has been a gold standard for treatment of biliary atresia was used. Life years gained was used as an index of health outcome for each strategy.

Table 16 shows the costs and health outcome per patient of LT and HP. The costs during the 6 year period in LT and HP were $164,600 and $22,300, respectively. Expected life years in LT and HP were 5.20 and 1.76. In the case of lifetime follow up, costs in both alternatives were $1,010,000 and $81,400. Expected life years gained were 63.28 and 6.41. At five year and lifetime follow-up, the cost-effectiveness (CE) ratios of LT in comparison with HP were $45,750 and $20,640 per life year gained, respectively (Table 17). The two-way sensitivity

Table 15   Cost-effectiveness analysis of living liver transplantation

Object: To compare efficiency of living liver transplantation for biliary atresia with hepatic portoenterostomy	
Study design	: CEA, Retrospective analysis
Standpoint	: Payer
Effectiveness	: Retrospective cohort study
Comparator	: Heapatic portoenterostomy
Outcome	: Life years gained
Costs	: Direct costs
Study period	: 6 years, lifetime
Efficiency	: Cost-effectiveness ratio ($/life year gained)
Discount rate	: 5% (costs and effectiveness)

Table 16   Cost and effectiveness of living liver transplantation

Therapy	Costs ($)		Expected life years	
	6 year	lifetime	6 year	lifetime
Conventional surgery	22,300	81,400	1.76	6.41
Liver transplantation	164,600	1,010,000	5.20	63.28

Table 17 Cost-effectiveness of living liver transplantation

Follow up	Incremental cost ($)	Incremental life years gained	Incremental cost-effectiveness ratio
6 year	135,000	2.95	$45,750
lifetime	314,400	15.24	$20,640

(Discount: 5% for cost and outcome)

analysis of incremental CE ratio according to discount rate for effectiveness and costs showed that it did not change notably.

These results show that living LT for biliary atresia is relatively efficient at the five year follow up. In addition, if costs and effectiveness are projected to lifetime, efficiency of LT is estimated to be increasing very rapidly. Although there are several differences in methods, costs and health outcomes, the results in this study are consistent with those reported before in the U.S.[29] and the Netherlands [30].

In Japan, the introduction and utilization of LT were not linked to any formal assessment in health policy. In this study, considerable potentiality for efficacy and efficiency of LT was observed. For the future, the effectiveness and efficiency of BMT need to be comprehensibly evaluated for appropriate and efficient utilization of LT.

CONCLUSION

These economic evaluations showed substantial possibilities for evaluating value for money of healthcare in Japan, to establish effective and efficient healthcare system. However, there are several fundamental obstacles to be overcome. Firstly, the government is required to make clear its strategies in using economic evaluation. Also, the strategies should promote incentives for healthcare professionals to supply efficient healthcare. Secondly, there are fundamental obstacles, closely related to the quality of economic evaluations, to be overcome. They include problems such as poor quality of randomized controlled trials, limited epidemiological data, limited cost data, and limited quality of life data. Although these obstacles are not easy to overcome, they must be dealt with successfully to incorporate economic evaluation into decision making for effective and efficient healthcare in Japan.

REFERENCE

1. Hisashige A (1997) Healthcare technology assessment and the challenge to pharmacoeconomics in Japan. Pharmacoeconomics 11:319-333
2. Gray JAM (1997) Evidence-based healthcare. Churchill Livingston, NY
3. OECD (1996) Health care reform. OECD, Paris
4. Burt RK, Deeg HJ, Lothian ST, Santos GW (1996) Bone marrow transplantation. Chapman & Hill, NY
5. Soutar RL, King DJ (1995) Bone marrow transplantation. BMJ, 310:31-36
6. Schweitzer SO, Scalzi CC (1981) The implication of cost-effectiveness analysis of medical technology, case study #6: the cost-effectiveness of bone marrow transplant therapy and its policy implications, Office of Technology Assessment, Congress of the United States, Washington DC
7. Magrath I (1995) Bone marrow transplantation for leukemia: a lame stalking horse for use of high-technology medical care. Lancet, 345:601-602
8. Welch HG, Larson EB (1989) Cost effectiveness of bone marrow transplantation in acute nonlympocytic leukemia. NEJM, 321:807-812
9. Drummond MF, Stoddart GL, Torrance GW (1987) Methods for the economic evaluation of health care programmes. Oxford Univ Press, Oxford.
10. Japan Adult Leukemia Study Goup (1993) Protocol of treatment for adult acute lymphatic leukemia

11. Ohnishi K, Ohno R, Tomonaga M, et al (1995) A randomized trial comparing interferon-with busulfan for newly diagnosed chronic myelogenous leukemia in chronic phase. Blood, 86:906-916

12. Henderson IG (1995) Paradigmatic shifts in the management of breast cancer. NEJM, 332:951-952

13. NIH consensus conference (1991) Treatment of early-stage breast cancer, JAMA, 265:391-395

14. Ganz PA (1992) Treatment options for breast cancer, beyond survival. NEJM, 326:1147-1149

15. Kieber GM, de Haes JCJM, de Velde CJH (1991) The impact of breast conserving treatment and mastectomy on the quality of life of early-stage breast cancer patients. J Clin Oncol, 9:1059-1070

16. Irvine D, Brown B, Crooks D, et al (1991) Psychosocial adjustment in women with breast cancer. Cancer, 67:1097-1117

17. Fallowfield LJ (1995) Assessment of quality of life in breast cancer. Acta Oncologica, 34:689-694

18. Dickersin K, Berlin JA (1992) Meta-analysis:State-of-the science. Epidem Review, 14:154-176

19. Beck JR, Pauker SG (1983) The Markov model in medical prognosis. Med Decision Making, 3:419-458

20. Hisashige A, Katayama T, Koike M, Mikasa H (1997) A clinical decision analysis of the choice of therapy for early breast cancer, Jpn J Breast Cancer, 12:3-12 (in Japanese)

21. Verhoef LCG, Stalpers LJA, Verbeek ALM, et al (1991) Breast-conserving treatment or mastectomy in early breast cancer. Eur J Cancer, 9:1132-1137

22. Coates A, Abraham S, Kay S, et al (1983) On the receiving end - patient perception of the side effects of cancer chemotherapy. Eur J Cancer Oncol, 19:203-208

23. O'Brien BJ, Rusthoven J, Rocchi A, et al (1993) Impact of chemotherapy-associated nausea and vomiting on patients' functional status and on costs: survey of five Canadian centres. Can Med Assoc, 149:296-316

24. Hesketh PJ, Gandara DR (1991) Serotonin antagonists, a new class of antiemetic agents. J Natl Can Inst, 83:613-620

25. Plosker GL, Milne RJ (1992) Ondansetron, a pharmacoeconomic and quality-of-life evaluation of its antiemetic activity in patients receiving cancer chemotherapy. Pharmacoeconomics, 2:285-304

26. Stiller CR (1988) High-tech medicine and the control of health care costs. Am J Med, 84:475-478

27. Michel BC, Van Hout BA, Bonsel GJ (1994) Assessing the benefits of transplant services. Bailliere's Clin Gastroenterol, 8:411-423

28. Matsui A, Sasaki N, Arakawa Y, et al (1993) Neonatal mass screening for biliary atresia. Screening, 2:201-209

29. Kankannpaa J (1987) Cost-effectiveness of liver transplantation, Transpl Proceedings, 19:3864-3866

30. Bonsel GJ, Klomopmaker IJ, Essik-Bot ML, et al (1990) Cost-effectiveness analysis of the Dutch liver transplantation programme. Transpl Proceedings, 22:1481-1484

Session Summary

Health Economics in Palliative Medicine

Shigeaki Yoshida[1], Kenji Eguchi[2]

[1] National Cancer Center Hospital East, Chiba, Japan
[2] National Shikoku Cancer Center, Matsuyama, Japan

The sessions began with a presentation by Associate Professor Thomas Smith, who focused on health economics for evaluating the cost of palliative care. He discussed the meaning of health economics research in several example of clinical situations, such as chemotherapy, home care, hospice care, and advanced directives. Findings of well-designed, randomized clinical trials will be useful for analyzing health economics in palliative medicine. He added that the results of health economics studies performed in different countries and different health care systems could be compared if important factors were properly identified with well-designed randomized trials. However, he warned that the results of health economic studies cannot be directly applied to individual patients or hospitals. In response to a question, Dr. Smith said that evaluating the quality of hospice care is difficult because of the value that patients place on their own lives. Any such evaluation would be subjective and depend on the satisfaction or patients and their families.

Dr. Smith said there were no established data on the relationship between advanced directive and cost savings in palliative medicine. He said it would be difficult to perform a randomized study of health economic comparing patients who had and had not established advanced directives during the early stage of their diseases. Furthermore, advanced directives established in the last few days before death would likely have little effect on the results of a study of the economics of care.

Professor Matthew Liang introduced general concepts of health economics research using examples of studies of patients with chronic rheumatoid diseases. There were questions about how to apply results of such studies to the decision-making of clinicians in different countries. Further discussion focused on how to evaluate and how to maintain the quality of medical practice with minimized cost, as cost minimization will be a major goal of this type of research. Two speakers answered that the consensus of respected practitioners and the perspectives of patients would be the best, most reliable way to judge the quality of medicine, although there are no universally valid method for evaluating the quality of medical practice. However, specialized committees and audits might also play a role in ensuring the quality of medical practice.

Professor Akinori Hisashige discussed the application of health economic research in liver transplantation for biliary atresia among neonates, bone marrow transplantation for leukemia in children, breast-conserving treatment for early breast cancer, and antiemetic treatment cancer patients receiving chemotherapy. In Japan, there are several fundamental obstacles to this type of research. These include a clear government strategy for health care, improvement in the quality of randomized controlled trials, limitations on acquisition of epidemiologic data, health care expense, and quality of life. Cooperation between clinicians and researchers is needed if clinically meaningful health economics research is to be performed.

Session VI

Quality of Life (QOL) Research

Chairpersons:
Thomas J. Smith and Yosuke Uchitomi

Quality of Life Evaluation in Chronic Illness Across Cultures

Sonya Eremenco, Kimberly Webster, and David Cella

Evanston Northwestern Healthcare
Northwestern University, Evanston, IL

SUMMARY. Quality of life (QOL) evaluation in chronic illness is a challenge even in one culture. Expanding that effort from our North American experience into Japanese language and culture has been an exciting and interesting challenge. Rigorous translation methods, followed by evaluation of measurement bias, will allow us to compare QOL in patients suffering from the same chronic diseases, who live in different cultures.

KEY WORDS: Quality of life, FACIT Measurement System, Multilingual translations

In the palliative treatment of chronic illness, attention must extend beyond disease and symptom control into an evaluation of overall quality of life (QOL). Effective appraisal of medical interventions deemed justifiable on the basis of providing comfort, palliation, or support of some kind, is important to demonstrating health outcomes and to improving the quality of patient care in a palliative setting. Evaluating the full spectrum of effects of such interventions increase the chance that real improvement in the overall functioning of the patient will be detected. It also helps inform clinical trial research of the true outcome of a given treatment. For these reasons, availability of standardized measures that allow for quality of life assessment and cross cultural comparison have become increasingly important to international clinical trial research with QOL endpoints. This paper reports on the newly revised version of one such measurement system, the Functional Assessment of Chronic Illness Therapy (FACIT) Measurement system, and on the multilingual translation of the Japanese version.

Quality of Life

The main dimensions of quality of life are physical, functional, mental and social [1-2]. The physical dimension refers to disease, symptoms, and treatment side effects. The functional dimension reflects primarily one's capabilities, role limitations and self care. The mental dimension includes emotional distress and positive emotional experiences. Finally, the social dimension relates to intimacy, sexuality and family relationships as well as the extended friendship network and the amount of support and help that people obtain from their social network.

The optimal quality of life evaluation program is one which is well-integrated with other clinical and laboratory data, and connected to a reporting mechanism that allows for self-correction of the treatment system. Efficient QOL assessment is that which asks the least number of questions to obtain needed precision. Questionnaires should be reliable and valid, and ideally, sensitive to targeted areas of change or treatment differences.

FACIT Measurement System

The FACIT system is a collection of QOL questionnaires targeted to the management of chronic illness. The term "FACIT' is a new one aimed to portray the expansion of the more familiar "FACT" series of questionnaires into other chronic illnesses and conditions, such as Multiple Sclerosis, HIV infection and Parkinson's Disease. The measurement system, under development since 1987, began with the creation of a generic CORE questionnaire called the Functional Assessment of Cancer Therapy-General (FACT-G). The FACT-G (now Version 4) is a 27-item compilation of general questions divided into four primary QOL domains: Physical Well-Being, Social/Family Well-Being, Emotional Well-Being, and Functional Well-Being. It is considered appropriate for use with patients with any form of cancer.

Validation of a core measure allowed for the evolution of multiple disease, treatment, condition, and non-cancer-specific subscales. FACIT scales are constructed to complement the FACT-G, addressing relevant disease-, treatment-, or condition-related issues not already covered in the general questionnaire. Each is intended to be as specific as necessary to capture the clinically-relevant problems associated with a given condition or symptom, yet general enough to allow for comparison across diseases, and extension, as appropriate, to other chronic medical conditions. The newest version of the FACIT Measurement System, Version 4, is designed to enhance clarity and precision of measurement without threatening its established reliability and validity. Formatting simplification, item-reduction, and rewording (standardizing items across scales) constitute the major areas of change. To facilitate the clinical utility of the FACIT system, new methods for computer acquisition, scoring and display of data will be available. In a palliative care setting, these additions and improvements will likely ease patient burden, expedite data collection and scoring, and further guide the clinician or researcher in meaningful interpretation.

Current implementation of the FACIT questionnaires range in use from Phase II and III clinical trials and other cancer related treatment evaluations, as an intervention tool in the clinical management of symptoms (both physical and psychological), and as an outcomes measure in health practice self studies. Equivalent foreign language versions of the FACIT questionnaires are now available in as many as 24 different languages, permitting cross-cultural comparisons of people from diverse backgrounds. Current and ongoing research with the FACIT questionnaires includes several projects designed to evaluate cross cultural equivalence, cross-instrument equivalence, and clinical significance.

The Japanese Experience

Current Japanese FACIT questionnaires include the FACT-G, -An (Anemia/fatigue), -B (breast cancer), -Bl (bladder cancer), -L (lung cancer), and –P (prostate cancer). These instruments have undergone a rigorous, well-established translation methodology which uses an iterative forward-backward translation sequence. Specifically, the steps are the following. First, native speakers of Japanese produce two independent forward translations from English into Japanese. In this case, a bilingual translator in Japan did one of the forward translations while a bilingual translator who has resided in the US for many years did the second. Next, a third independent bilingual translator, also a native speaker of Japanese, reconciled the two forward translations, or chose the better of the two item by item. In some cases, it was necessary for the reconciler to make modifications to the existing translations or combine them. Next, a native English speaker, ideally from the United States, who is fluent in Japanese, back-translated from the Japanese reconciled version. Then, three bilingual experts reviewed the entire translation process, taking into consideration comments made by the Translation Coordinating Team. Once all reviews were complete, Mr. Hiro Tsuchiya compiled them and selected the final version for testing. The last step in the process is pre-testing, in which native speaking patients answer the questionnaire and then participate in a short interview to give feedback to improve the questionnaire.

The Japanese version of the FACT-G, L and Anemia was initially tested with lung cancer patients in Japan, almost all of whom were experiencing fatigue or anemia as a result of their disease or treatment. Because of difficulties in understanding some of the translations and the concepts in these items, the questionnaire was revised and re-tested with another set of Japanese-speaking lung cancer patients. Dr. Kunihiko Kobayashi was instrumental in the development of these first three scales and is halfway through a validation study using them. During this process, the translation of the Breast cancer scale was begun with the participation of Dr. Kojiro Shimozuma, and incorporated some of the issues that arose during the previous translation effort. After completion of the translation of the FACT-B, it was successfully tested with breast cancer patients in Japan, and is now considered trial ready. The last phase of the translation process began with the bladder and prostate cancer subscales, the testing of which was recently completed in Version 4 format. These last two scales incorporated significant input from the researchers including Miyuki Niimi, R.N., in Japan, as a way of bridging the cultural and linguistic gaps between the US and Japan. In addition, Dr. Hiroko Arioka has developed a scale for Bronchial Asthma using the FACIT model which will accompany the FACT-G in an upcoming validation project.

The adaptation of the FACIT system for use in Japan presented great challenges to addressing cultural differences between Eastern and Western societies in addition to linguistic differences inherent in translation. One of the major issues that arose early in the translation process was the difference in the medical system in Japan and in the relationship between doctor and patient. In the US, doctors are legally obligated to inform the patient of his or her diagnosis so that the patient may make treatment-related decisions with the advice of the doctor. In contrast, in Japan, the doctor traditionally does not give the patient the diagnosis of cancer, but instead informs the family who then agree on the best course of treatment with the doctor. It is then up to the family to inform the patient about the diagnosis if they so choose. Several translators felt that it would be inappropriate to give Japanese patients a questionnaire like the FACT when they often are not informed that they have cancer.

Another issue that was addressed by the translators was the difference in sentence structure between Japanese and English. Almost all of the original FACT items begin with "I" to reflect the patient's point of view. In Japanese, the pronoun "I" is not used in the questionnaire but understood by the context of the question. Despite this omission, it seems that patients do not feel comfortable revealing their personal feelings, even in the impersonal format of circling numbers on the questionnaire. They feel that they must answer truthfully, and would rather leave items blank than answer inaccurately.

Quality of life measurement often includes both negatively and positively stated items, primarily to avoid response set. In Japanese, when items are negatively stated, the negative or "no" comes at the end of the sentence regardless of how it is worded in English. This may account for the reason patients continue to have difficulty with changes in direction of item wording (positive vs. negative) that are typical in psychometric questionnaires. They term this a "change in polarity" and find it quite disconcerting. Experience thus far has shown that they would prefer the response choice "0" to always indicate a bad condition and the response choice "4" to always indicate a good condition. This would help to reduce their confusion. Psychometric analysis often revealed that items that were the reverse polarity from the majority of other items in a particular subscale, had negative or very low correlations with the subscale. While we could not make the polarity uniform, we decided that it would be necessary to add a line to the instructions to let patients know that the polarity might change and not to expect consistency.

The next major difference related to the role of the family and larger society in the patient's quality of life. We discovered in our first testing that patients do not consider friends and neighbors to be as important to their quality of life as their family. In some cases, this resulted in a patient leaving items referring to friends and family blank because they felt that they could not identify with the concept of the importance of friends and neighbors to their quality of life and did not want to lie on the questionnaire. Differences in family structure also became apparent. Patients were reluctant to single out their spouse or partner as their primary source of support. Instead, they felt that it was important to include an item about other family members. The item that caused the most difficulty was item GP3, in English "Because of my physical condition, I have trouble meeting the needs of my family". While this item could be translated literally, it was meaningless to the patient. After analyzing patient comments on this question, and consultations with Dr. Kobayashi, it was determined that the issue of greater concern is that patients feel like a burden to their families, and this has a negative effect on their quality of life. Therefore, item GP3 in Japanese now reads: "I feel that I have become a burden to my family because of my physical condition" and as such has been much more acceptable to patients. Other changes included adding two additional family centered items to test whether these were more relevant to the patients. We added: "I feel close to my family" and "My family is doing well despite my illness" for the purpose of assessing if a more family-oriented subscale would produce a stronger Social/Family Well-Being scale.

Two problematic issues of major concern to Japanese patients are sexuality and mortality. Japanese patients, whether male or female, do not like to answer questions about their sexuality. We are told that it is not culturally appropriate to ask such a question, and that patients feel shame when answering them. However, most of them do answer the questions out of a desire to please the doctor or interviewer who has asked them to participate in the testing. In order to be sensitive to this cultural difference, we attempted to soften the sexuality-related questions as much as possible. In fact, on the FACT-B, we substituted the phrase "I feel attractive as a woman" for the English item "I feel sexually attractive" because of sensitivity to seeing the word "sex" on paper. Similar problems arose with the item GE4 "I worry about dying". Patients consistently mention how they do not wish to even see the character for death in print. It appears that just thinking about death or reading the word can induce anxiety that it may happen. This is also problematic when the patient may not know that his or her illness is cancer, instead of an ulcer or some other benign illness. While we in the West feel that knowledge is important for the patient to be able to confront and overcome the illness, it may be that in other cultures, ignorance is truly bliss, and the patient is protected by not knowing the diagnosis and severity of the illness.

A final linguistic issue that was difficult to resolve related to the item response categories such as "not at all" and "very much so". Japanese patients found them too vague in the early rounds of testing, partly due to the tendency of the Japanese language to be less specific. We resolved the problem by adding more context to the response categories so that they would be more relevant to the items that they were intended to answer. Thus, the response categories now read "not at all applicable, a little bit applicable, somewhat applicable, quite a bit applicable, very much applicable". While the redundancy may seem unnecessary in English, it seems vital in Japanese to keep the patient focused on the responses. This addition to the response categories seems to have resolved some of the difficulties with patient comprehension of certain items.

All of the pre-testing was done with patient samples of 10-15 patients per subscale. At this time, validation studies are underway for the FACT-L with lung cancer patients and FACT-B with breast cancer patients to assess the QOL impact of different treatment arms for each type of cancer. With larger data sets, we will be able to assess and compare QOL of Japanese breast and lung cancer patients with similar patients in US trials, expanding possibilities for cross-cultural comparisons.

REFERENCES

1. Cella DF, Tulsky DS, Gray G, et al: The Functional Assessment of Cancer Therapy (FACT) Scale: Development and validation of the general measure. *Journal of Clinical Oncology* 11(3):570-579, 1993.

2. Cella DF & Bonomi AE: Measuring quality of life today: 1995 update. *Oncology* 9(11):47-60, 1995.

QUALITY OF LIFE IN PALLIATIVE MEDICINE: CURRENT STATUS AND PROBLEMS OF QOL RESEARCH IN JAPAN

Kunihiko Ishitani, M.D., Department of Internal Medicine, Higashi Sapporo Hospital, Sapporo, Japan

SUMMARY. In 1996 a multicenter collaborative study was conducted throughout Japan on the current status of cancer patients who were being cared for at home. In the study, the main patient outcome measure was the quality of life (QOL). Prior to the study, instruments for assessment of the QOL were investigated. Comparison and evaluation of two types of authorized multidimensional QOL measure and a single QOL measure showed good correlation between the three measures. As a result, the single QOL measure was employed for the research. The QOL scores of 208 registered patient cases when transferred to home care showed a biphasic distribution. The patients who scored in the lower QOL range were predominantly 69 years or younger, while those in the higher QOL range were mostly 70 years or older. Anxiety was a key factor in the QOL of the patients aged 69 or younger, whereas a depressed mood was a key factor in the QOL of the patients aged 70 years or older. These findings confirm the importance of psychiatric and psychological care to home cancer care. The spiritual domain of QOL in palliative medicine is a controversial issue. A single QOL measure is believed to be practical for clinical studies which require simplicity, and this measure must include the spiritual domain.

KEY WORDS: Quality of life (QOL), Palliative Medicine, QOL assessment instrument, Home cancer care, Spiritual problem

INTRODUCTION

Today, a good QOL is the principal goal even in general oncology [1] . On the other hand, in 1989, the World Health Organization directed the following statement to the entire world: "The primary goal of palliative care is to optimize the QOL of patients with advanced incurable illness through control of physical symptoms and through attention to the patient's psychological, social and spiritual needs." [2] In spite of this pronouncement, QOL research in the field of palliative medicine remains surprisingly scanty at present. There are only a few recent research efforts which, on the basis of evidence-based medicine, are able to withstand statistical evaluation [3-7] . In reality, it can be thought that research as evidence-based medicine in the field of palliative medicine is still rare throughout the world. In Japan, QOL research has a history of about 20 years in the field of general oncology. The approaches taken are basically the same as those applied in other countries [8] . However, in palliative medicine, hardly any QOL clinical research has been carried out which is capable of withstanding statistical evaluation. Between January of 1996 and March of 1997, in cooperation with 22 medical care institutions throughout Japan, we carried out a questionnaire survey of 208 advanced cancer patients who were being cared for at home. Measurement of the QOL was employed as the main outcome measure. This multicenter collaborative study of advanced cancer patients being treated at home was not carried out with the primary objective of performing QOL research, but some information was obtained.

QOL assessment as the main outcome measure of research on home cancer care

In Japan, almost all cancer patients have conventionally been treated in hospitals, and only recently has there finally been recognition of the need for at-home cancer care. However, at present home care for cancer patients remains very limited in scale, and almost all of those cases are handled as volunteer activities of the medical facility. Whether high-tech home care or traditional home care (that is, hospice home care), the content of the care is based on experience, and there has still been no establishment of standards founded on evidence-based medicine. The objective of research which requested by the Japanese Foundation for Multidisciplinary Treatment of Cancer was development of a rational system for home cancer care. As concrete objectives, social science research has been started in relation to (1) investigation of patient satisfaction with home cancer care, and elucidation of the various factors which influence that satisfaction, and (2) elucidation of the functions of each medical care giver in home cancer care and cooperation among them. A committee was established with the objective of studying research design. That committee first discussed the adoption of QOL assessment for determining the level of patient satisfaction and also the instrument to be used for QOL assessment.

In our hospital, we perform QOL assessment by means of a categorical measure which we developed ourselves, with guaranteed reliability and validity (Table 1) [8]. During the past 10 years, we have routinely performed QOL assessment once every 2 weeks for more than 5,000 cancer patients treated at our hospital. We have employed QOL assessment for monitoring of the quality of care and as material for various QOL research. When we carry out our QOL assessment, which is based on 10 items, we also employ a single-scale evaluation (Table 2) for assessment of the global QOL [9] . The total point score with the QOL measure used by our hospital and the single-scale measure showed good correlation, with a coefficient of correlation of −0.681. In addition, it can be expected that the persons mainly responsible for carrying out this research on home cancer care are the nurses, while most of the patients can be expected to be advanced cancer patients. Under these circumstances, it will be desirable for the instrument to have simplicity [10] . Therefore, on the basis of our experience, the committee proposed that the single-scale measure be employed as the main outcome measure of this research.

Table 1. Higashi-Sapporo Hospital QOL measure
QUALITY OF LIFE QUESTIONNAIRE FOR SELF-ASSESSMENT

1. How is your appetite?
   1) good
   2) fair
   3) poor
   4) I don't eat at all.

2. How do you feel?
   1) very good
   2) fair
   3) bad
   4) very bad

3. How well do you sleep?
   1) very well
   2) fairly well
   3) not very well
   4) I don't sleep at all.

4. How much pain do you feel?
   1) none
   2) Some, but it's not so bad.
   3) It's bad, but I can tolerate it.
   4) It's almost intolerable.

5. Do you experience nausea or vomiting?
   1) No.
   2) Some, but it's not so bad.
   3) They are bad, but I can tolerate them.
   4) They are almost intolerable.

6. Are you experiencing any other symptoms?
   1) No
   2) Some symptoms, but not so bad.
   3) They are bad, but I can tolerate them.
   4) They are almost intolerable.

   In the cases of answers 2)-4) above, describe the symptoms:

7. How is your mood?
   1) very good
   2) fair
   3) some anxiety
   4) much anxiety

8. Are you able to enjoy TV, radio, books, etc?
   1) very much
   2) somewhat
   3) not very much
   4) not at all

9. Are you satisfied with your relationships with your doctors and nurses?
   1) very much
   2) yes
   3) somewhat dissatisfied
   4) dissatisfied

10. How is your daily life? For inpatients (life in the hospital)
    1) I am able to move about freely.
    2) I do not need any assistance with things around me or to walk.
    3) I frequently need assistance with things around me and to walk.
    4) I am bedridden, so I always need help.

Table 2. Single-scale evaluation

How would you rate your general feeling of well-being today?

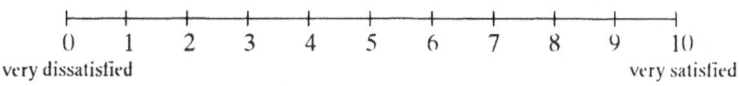

The committee also proposed that the relationships of the single-scale measure to other QOL instruments be investigated. Accordingly, an analysis was made of the relationship of the single-scale measure with the Kurihara QOL measure (Table 3) [11] . The Kurihara QOL measure was prepared by the QOL Working Group of the Ministry of Health and Welfare, which was headed by Prof. Kurihara of Showa University. The Kurihara QOL measure is comprised of 22 questions which the patients answer, and this is the only QOL measure to be officially authorized in Japan. The Kurihara QOL measure employs a face scale for assessment of the global QOL. Of course, the reliability, validity, etc., of this questionnaire have been statistically confirmed. We employed both of these QOL assessment instruments to measure the QOL in 81 randomly selected cancer patients in various stages of disease treated in Higashi Sapporo Hospital. We then analyzed the results with both instruments to determine the degree of their correlation. The correlation coefficient between the single-scale measure and the total score with the Kurihara QOL measure was 0.630. When we looked at the correlation coefficients for each of the domains, we found that the values were 0.62 for the psychological state, 0.59 for the social function and 0.58 for the face scale (Table 4, 5). Table 6 compiles the data showing the change in the single-scale measure and Kurihara QOL measure total point scores with the passage of time from the initial assessment to one month later. Three or more assessments were able to be made for 43 of the 81 cancer patients who were the subjects of this study. Calculation of the correlation coefficient of the difference between the initial assessment and the assessment after one month with each of the instruments gave a value of 0.66. That is, both of these assessment instruments show similar patterns of change with the passage of time. We conclude that the single-scale measure is a reliable method for evaluating the temporal change in the global QOL of cancer patients.

These results thus proved that the single-scale measure is an effective assessment instrument for achieving a unified or overall understanding of the QOL of cancer patients [12]. Accordingly, the single-scale measure has been adopted as the main outcome measure for evaluation of home care of cancer patients.

Table 3. Kurihara-QOL Measure

Questionnaire

This questionnaire will help us understand your current condition.

Please circle the number that best describes your condition in the past few days. (This information will remain strictly confidential and will not in any way affect your therapy. Please answer exactly the way you feel.)

1. How well were you able to accomplish your daily activities ?

    5   4   3   2   1
    Not at all   Fully accomplished

2. How often were you able to go out without help ?

    5   4   3   2   1
    Not at all   Did not need any help at all

3. Were you able to take a half-hour walk ?

    5   4   3   2   1
    Not at all   Without any problem

4. Did you feel any difficulty walking even a short distance ?

    5   4   3   2   1
    Did not have any problem   Very much

5. Were you able to walk up and down the stairs ?

    5   4   3   2   1
    Not at all   Yes, no problem

6. Were you able to take a bath by yourself ?

    5   4   3   2   1
    Not at all   Yes, without any help

7. How well did you feel ?

    5   4   3   2   1
    Very poor   Very well

8. Did you have a good appetite ?

    5   4   3   2   1
    Not at all   Very much

9. Did you enjoy your meals ?

    5   4   3   2   1
    Not at all   Very much

10. Did you experience any vomiting ?

    5   4   3   2   1
    None   Very often

11. Did you lose any weight ?

    5   4   3   2   1
    No, I have rather gained weight   Yes

12. Did you sleep well ?

    5   4   3   2   1
    Not at all   Very well

13. Were you able to devote yourself to (become enthusiastic about) something ?

    5   4   3   2   1
    Not at all   Very much

14. How well were you able to deal with your stress ?

    5   4   3   2   1
    Not at all   Very well

15. Did you feel you could not concentrate on anything ?

    5   4   3   2   1
    Yes, very much   Not at all

16. Did you get any encouragement from something/somebody you believe/trust (e.g., family, friends, religion, hobby) ?

    5   4   3   2   1
    Not at all   Very well

17. Did you worry about your disease ?

    5   4   3   2   1
    Not at all   Very much

18. Did you have any problem dealing with people outside your family ?

    5   4   3   2   1
    No problem   Very much

19. Did you think your family was troubled by your getting treatment ?

    5   4   3   2   1
    Not at all   Very much

20. Do you worry about your social life in the future ?

    5   4   3   2   1
    Not at all   Very much

21. How much do you worry about the financial burden of your treatment ?

    5   4   3   2   1
    Not at all   Very much

22. Please circle the number of the face that best fits your feelings in the past few days.

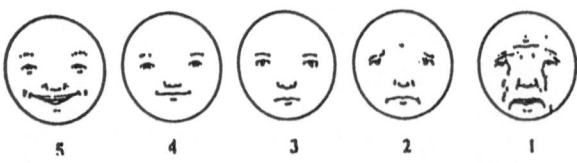

    5   4   3   2   1

Table 4. Correlation coefficients between the single-scale measure and
each of the domains of the Kurihara QOL measure

Physical activity (Q1~6)		0.45
Somatic sensation (Q7-11)	0.37	
Psychological state (Q12-16)	0.62	
Social function (Q17-21)	0.59	
Face scale (Q22)	0.58	
Total score (Q1~22)		0.63

Table 5. Correlation coefficients between each of the measures

	1	2	3
1. Single-scale	1.000		
2. Kurihara-QOL	0.630	1.000	
3. Higashi Sapporo Hospital-QOL	-0.681	-0.695	1.000

Table 6. Change in single-scale measure and the total point score of the
Kurihara QOL measure with passage of time

	Initial	After 1 Month
Single-scale Measure		
Mean	5.6	6.0
Median	5.0	6.0
S.D.	2.8	2.4
Kurihara QOL Measure		
Mean	69.6	72.8
Median	68.0	72.0
S.D.	17.2	16.5

Outlines of the research for home cancer care

The items included in the assessment table were prepared by the committee for use in the performance of surveys of the actual status of multicenter collaborative home cancer care studies. The assessment is performed with the passage of time, starting with when the patient returns home and then every 2 weeks thereafter, continuing until the patient dies at home or is readmitted to the hospital. The assessment items consist of a total of 34 patient outcomes, including physical symptoms, psychological symptoms, and so forth. Each item is evaluated using a scale having 4 levels. The single-scale measure is also used to assess the QOL at the same time. The reliability of this assessment table was investigated by having two nurses carry out assessment of the same patients at the same times and then determining the ratio of agreement for each item. The results showed that the values for the ratio of agreement were distributed in the range of 0.83 to 1.0, and the values for Cohen's agreement constant K were also similar. Thus, the reliability of this assessment table was confirmed.

22 institutions participated in the multicenter collaborative study of advanced cancer patients, and 10 of those facilities had hospice/palliative care units. From January of 1996 through March of 1997, 208 cancer patients were registered. (Table 7)   It is seen that the mean age was 67 years. The largest age subgroup was the patients in their seventies, who represented 32.7% of the total, and the second largest subgroup was patients in their sixties, representing 26.9% of the total. There was no difference in the number of registered patients as a function of whether or not the institution had a hospice/palliative care unit. The objective of almost all of the patients was to obtain palliative care.

Table 7. Patient background factors in home care study

Total No. of Cases	208	
Male:Female Ratio	97 : 111	
Mean Age (yr)	67.0 (median: 68; SD±13.9)	
Type of Cancer		
Gastric	47	(22.6%)
Colon	38	(18.3%)
Lung	29	(13.9%)
Pancreatic	18	(8.7%)
Gall bladder	17	(8.2%)
Liver	12	(5.8%)
Breast	14	(6.7%)
Prostate	10	(4.8%)
Esophageal	9	(4.3%)
Gynecological	8	(3.8%)
Head and neck	7	(3.4%)
Other	9	(4.4%)

Investigation of Patients' QOL in home care studies

Fig. 1 shows a plot of the distribution of QOL scores at the time of transfer to home care. There was thus an overall tendency for many of the patients to have a comparatively good QOL. That is, patients with a good QOL were the targets of home care. In addition, it can be seen from the graph that the QOL score shows a biphasic distribution, with peaks at scores of 5 and 8. We carried out an analysis of the data to determine the meaning and origin of this biphasic distribution of the QOL score in the cancer patients. No correlations were found with the patient's sex, type of cancer, whether or not the patient had been informed of the disease, or the severity of the symptoms. However, when we investigated the patients as two age subgroups, with 70 years as the cut-off, we found a correlation. That is, the elderly patients aged 70 years or more showed a distribution which was shifted to a high QOL score, whereas the younger patients aged 69 years or less were distributed in the lower QOL score range. (Fig. 2) These results were also found to show a statistically significant difference. We thus surmised that the biphasic distribution of the QOL score in the cancer patients was primarily due to the effect of age.

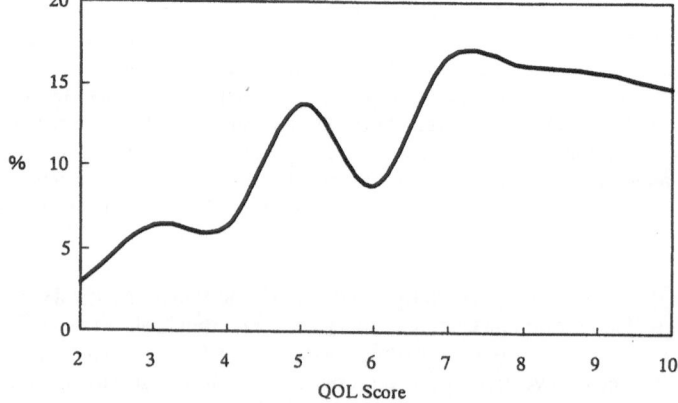

Fig. 1 Distribution of QOL scores at time of transfer to home care

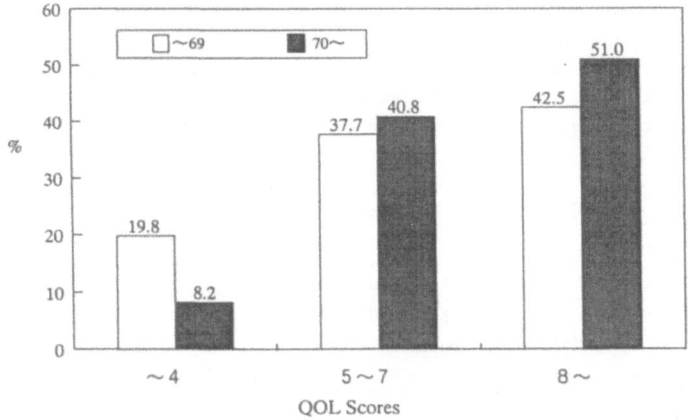

Fig. 2 Distribution of QOL scores as function of patient age

We investigated the change in the QOL as a function of time. The studied population consisted of 96 cases who had exceeded 6 weeks in home cancer care. The QOL was improved after 6 weeks in 45% of the patients, whereas it was aggravated in 33% (Fig. 3). Of course, in many of the patients the disease followed the usual course of progression, but in spite of that fact the QOL was maintained.

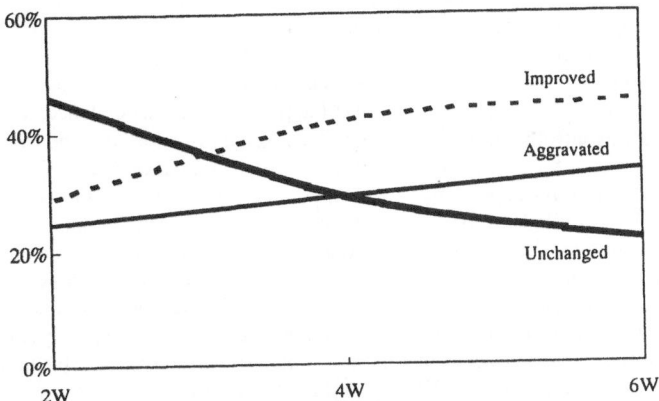

Fig. 3 Change in QOL score with passage of time

The factors influencing the QOL in these cancer patients were investigated by determining the Spearman correlation coefficients for each of the 34 items making up the patient outcomes in the assessment table (Table 8). It is seen that, in the younger (69 years old or less) patient group, the QOL score showed strong correlations with the items anxiety, QOL of the family member (assessed using the same single-scale measure as used for the QOL of the patient) and insomnia. In the older (at least 70 years old) patient group, a depressed mood showed a strong correlation with the QOL score. When the change in anxiety was looked at over a period of 6 weeks, the younger patient group was found to include a large number of patients who had anxiety from the time of the start of home cancer care, and there was a subsequent tendency for the anxiety to increase slightly. On the other hand, in the older group of patients aged 70 years or more, 56.5% of the patients had no anxiety at the time of the start of home cancer care, and thereafter there was a slight increase in anxiety, but the tendency was weak. The difference between the two patient groups was statistically significant.

The importance of psychiatric and psychological care to home cancer care has been pointed out. However, what is the origin of home cancer care patients' anxiety? We surmise that this will become clear in the course of providing psychiatric and psychological care to the individual patients [13]. When carrying out QOL surveys and home care, the existence or absence of anxiety will be revealed by the assessment, thereby achieving the objective of the assessment.

Table 8. Factors related to QOL

≦69 Years Old		≧70 Years Old	
Anxiety	-0.739	Depressed mood	-0.577
QOL of family member	0.658	QOL of family member	0.479
Insomnia	-0.558	Anxiety	-0.472
General fatigue	-0.480		

DISUCUSSION

The existence of a psychological state of anxiety exerted a strong influence on the difference in the QOL score distribution between patients younger than 70 years old and patients aged 70 years or more. Our analysis of the data generated for the 208 investigated cases is still incomplete, but it can at least be stated that no clear correlation has been found between the physical condition of the cancer patients and the QOL score distribution. In addition, a later section deals with the relationship between the QOL score distribution and notification of the disease, but it is noted here that more of the patients in the younger group had been told the truth about their disease [14]. The difference between the two age groups above and below 70 years of age has some meaning in Japan. That is, the defeat of Japan in World War Two caused a major change in the culture of Japan. Prior to World War Two, Japanese had lived their lives on a moral basis of mutual dependence, whereas after the defeat in the war there was introduction of Western values based on autonomy and individualism, and this teaching continues today. What this means is that the older generation above 70 years of age was raised on the morality of mutual dependence and experienced the war, leaving them more religious than the younger generation below 70 years of age. Conversely, the younger generation lives their lives with autonomy as the standard, and they are still socially and professionally active. My personal opinion is that the stronger tendency for anxiety in the younger patient group is due to this cultural difference from the older patient group. Stated in a different way, autonomy is a hard path to follow when you know the truth about your disease and must make decisions yourself about your disease, treatment and life. This concept of the importance of differences in spiritual/psychological culture will probably become a theme for QOL research in the future.

The Kurihara QOL measure was originally developed as an outcome measure for randomized clinical trials on anticancer agents. However, at present, this QOL measure is being employed in various clinical situations as a measure of the outcome of cancer therapy as a whole. The Higashi Sapporo Hospital QOL measure was initially developed primarily for use in patients with advanced/recurrent/terminal cancer, and it is being used all around Japan. In relation to hospice and palliative care, pertinent papers in this field always point out the need to add a spiritual or existential domain to the QOL questionnaire [15]. However, there have been very few published papers which set forth concrete questions relating to the spiritual or existential domain, and even fewer papers have dealt with the reliability and rationality of such questions. Recently, there has been an approach in which the spiritual problem is considered to mean a search for meaning and is placed in the sphere of psycho-social problems [5,16]. However, in Japan, most QOL researchers do not pay much attention to the spiritual problem. In fact, we can probably even say that the most common attitude is denial of the existence of a spiritual problem. Does spiritual distress in fact exist? If it does, then how do we evaluate it? However, if we assume that spiritual distress does indeed exist, why would it be special to cancer patients? Wouldn't it exist for all living people? In that case, shouldn't it be handled on a broader social scale, not just in the medical care field? It is possible to imagine that spiritual distress might be involved in the anxiety felt by cancer patients. Assuming that it is, medical personnel should, for the time being, use the single-scale measure to achieve an understanding of spiritual distress in each patient.

REFERENCES

1. American Society of Clinical Oncology (1996) Outcomes of cancer treatment for technology assessment and cancer treatment guidelines. J Clin Oncol 14:671-679
2. WHO Expert Committee on Cancer Pain Relief and Active Supportive Care (1990) Cancer pain relief and palliative care. WHO Technical Report Series No.804
3. Bruera E, Kuhean N, Miller MJ, Selmser P, MacMillan K (1991) The Edmonton symptom assessment system (ESAS): A simple method for the assessment of palliative care patients. J Palliat Care 7:6-9
4. Higginson I, McCarthy M (1993) Validity of the support team assessment schedule: do staffs' ratings reflect those made by patients or their families? Palliat Med 7:219-228
5. McMillian SC, Mahon M (1994) Measuring quality of life in hospice patients using a newly developed Hospice Quality of Life Index. Qual Life Res 3: 437-447
6. Ellershaw JE, Peat SJ, Boys LC (1995) Assessing the effectiveness of a hospital palliative care team. Palliat Med 9: 145-152
7. Cohen SR, Mount BM, Strobel MG, Bui F (1995) The McGill quality of life questionnaire: a measure of quality of life appropriate for people with advanced disease. A preliminary study of validity and acceptability.
8. Ishitani K (1991) Quality of life and cancer pain relief. Proc. WHO Workshop on Cancer Pain Relief and Quality of Life, Saitama Cancer Center, Shalom, Tokyo, pp 64-72
9. Kawamata M, Ishitani K, Ishikawa K, Sasaki H, Ota K, Omote K, Namiki A (1996) Comparison between celiac plexus block and morphine treatment on quality of life in patients with pancreatic cancer pain. Pain 64: 597-602
10. Richards MA (1997) Quality of life: the main outcome measure of palliative care. Palliat Med 11: 89-92
11. Kurihara M, Shimizu H, Tsuboi K, Kobayashi K, Murakami M, Eguchi K, Shimozuma K (in press) The Development of Quality of Life Questionaire in Japan. Psycho-Oncol.
12. Donnelly S, Walsh D (1996) Quality of life assessment in advanced cancer. Palliat Med 10: 275-283
13. Minagawa H, Uchitomi Y, Yamawaki S, Ishitani K (1996) Psychiatric morbidity in terminally ill cancer patients. Cancer 78: 1131-1137
14. Hamaguchi K, Ishigaki Y, Ishitani K (1997) Patients' perceptions of palliation in Japan. Proc. International Symposium on Current Perspectives and Future Directions in Palliative Medicine. Springer-Verlag Tokyo, Inc.
15. Ahmedzai S (1990) Measuring quality of life in hospice care. Oncol 4:115-119
16. Walten T (1997) The ideology and organization of spiritual care: three approaches. Palliat Med 11: 21-30

Quality of Life (QOL) Research

Yosuke Uchitomi

Chief, Psycho-Oncology Division, National Cancer Center Research East
6-5-1, Kashiwanoha, Kashiwa 277, Japan

Quality of Life has now been accepted as the universal concepts in Clinical Oncology as well as Palliative Medicine. Some researchers have spearheaded research to understand how cultures and health care system impact on patient's QOL. Research also explores and seeks to understand nuclear parts of QOL which is similar in all patients, irrespective of the social cultural context. In this session, methodological issues in QOL research including cross cultural issues have been discussed.

Dr. Cella introduced the original Measurement System called "Functional Assessment of Chronic Illness Therapy (FACIT)" for an international clinical trial research as QOL endpoints, which he and his colleagues have developed since 10 years ago. The System consisted of general core questionnaire with 29 items, called "Functional Assessment of Cancer Therapy-General version (FACT-G)" and specific questionnaires for various cancer sites, treatments, symptoms, respectively. FACIT are now available in as many as 24 different language, allowing researchers to compare cross cultural issues in chronic illness including cancer. He also presented the experience with Japanese researchers and linguist of the adaptation of the FACIT system for use in Japan with cultural and linguistic differences. In the discussion time, some audience questioned why the change of QOL after the Clinical Trial could predict survival time in Clinical Trial of anti-cancer drugs, how Japanese vcancer patients could be evaluated without their diagnose disclosed. Dr. Cella did not answer
exactly, but again stressed on the core QOL with additional items to bridge the cultural gap in Clinical Oncology as well as Palliative Medicine.

Dr. Ishitani pointed out critical issues in QOL research in Palliative Care setting, presenting the recent findings on QOL in caring for terminally ill cancer patients at home from multi-institutional studies in Japan. In their study, they demonstrated high correlation between single item- measured global QOL scale and Kurihara 22 item-QOL scale developed in Japan. One of the audience commented the correlation is extremely high. Dr. Ishitani did not tell exactly, but emphasized only one single item-measured global QOL scale is important in caring for terminally ill patients, who are physically exhausted. And he also mentioned some important issues in QOL research; 1) Can we evaluate the incompetent patients (e.g., delirium, dementia...)? 2) How we can manage the QOL of the patients without their diagnosis given? Since most Eastern countries do not disclose the truth. 3) How we can evaluate the spiritual and existential aspects of QOL? Dr. Cella commented the last issues, that adding specific items for spiritual dimensions of QOL in the cultural context should be considered. Finally, Dr. Smith summarized the session and emphasized the importance of awareness of QOL in advanced and terminally-ill patients, and evidence-based QOL research in Palliative Medicine.

Session VII

Patient Education and Ethics

Chairpersons:
Harvey M. Chochinov and Makoto Aoki

Future Detectors and Sites

COMPLEMENTARY MEDICINE

Stephen C. Schimpff, M.D.

Executive Vice President, University of Maryland Medical System, 22 South Greene Street, Baltimore, MD 21201, USA

SUMMARY. Complementary medicine has a clear role in palliative care of cancer and AIDS. If one is to follow a holistic approach to medical care, one in which the focus is on healing and not just an attempt at cure of the underlying disease, then complementary medicine techniques are clearly appropriate. True, they have not received the type of scientific validation that might be desirable, but to the extent that the patient finds relief and has an improved quality of life as a result of these techniques, then the use of complementary techniques is clearly valid and appropriate. Furthermore, it is clear that patients use complementary approaches with or without their doctor's knowledge or recommendation, and it therefore behooves physicians to recognize that their patients may well be visiting complementary medical practitioners. That being the case, it is better that physician and complementary medicine practitioner work together as a team, understanding what each team member can add to the overall care and healing of the patient.

KEY WORDS: Holistic medicine, complementary medicine, acupuncture, mind-body medicine, massage, herbal therapies.

TOWARD A HOLISTIC MODEL OF MEDICINE

The fundamental goals of Medicine are cure, promoting health, preventing illness and injury, restoring functional capacity, avoiding premature death, relieving suffering, and caring for those who cannot be cured. American medicine and indeed that of most countries which have a predominance of "science-based medicine," or what I will term "conventional medicine," focuses primarily on only the first of these goals, namely, cure. Ellen Fox, in a recent editorial of the Journal of the American Medical Association [1] speaks of the predominance of the curative model of medical care and defines this as a model focused on eradication of the cause of illness or disease but which tends not to focus on the other goals of medicine referred to above. The curative model by its very nature carries with it certain attitudes, assumptions and values. Among them is an analytic and rationalistic approach to medicine where the object of the practitioner's attention is not the patient but the disease. The symptoms are clues to diagnosis but, in and of themselves, are not the object of treatment. Since cure is contingent upon diagnosis and then therapy, the practitioner of conventional medicine is highly invested in the scientific approach. Thus, the physician values scientifically based data over all others. For example, there is a high focus on and attention to the results of laboratory tests, radiologic studies and a lesser appreciation for the subjective elements of the history. Another attitude is that psychological factors which arise through the history are regarded as rather trivial despite the fact that these psychological factors may play a large component in determining the patients quality of life. As a result, facts become differentiated from feelings and the body becomes differentiated from the mind. We frequently hear on morning rounds "the gallbladder in room 706" rather than "the lady in room 706 who has symptoms which suggest gallbladder disease." In like manner, practitioners tend to perceive a patient in terms of component parts rather than as a total person. Finally and perhaps most importantly, the curative model conflicts with the notion of a "good death." To the physician, death is the ultimate failure and the patient or the patient's disease ends up being labeled as "untreatable." The result, Dr. Fox suggests, is a neglect of palliative care [1].

Since death is seen as a medical failure, it sends a message to medical students and residents in a sense of a "hidden curriculum." This undermines the attitudes that form the basis for compassion and effective care of the dying [2]. This focus on cure as the critical goal of medicine and with it the neglect of palliative care drives the resident in training, who feels the need to be as efficient as possible, to "turf" psychosocial tasks, to avoid intimacy with patients and family, to embrace hierarchical structures and to float above commitment [3]. The physician in training tends to believe that psychosocial activities with patients is less important or to the extent that they are important at all can be taken care of by other members of the health care team. The avoidance of intimacy comes with the resident's (and later the practicing physician's) inability to be intimate with the patient because of his or her own sense of inadequacy if not failure at the inability to cure the disease. This also leads to the creation of hierarchical structures of the medical team with the physician as superior and the one who deals with the "truly important" issues related to cure whereas "lower" individuals within the hierarchy, such as nurses, social workers, et al. can deal with the compassionate aspect of care. The result is that the team is not made up of individuals all respected equally for their expertise, actions and commitment but rather as those who are more or less important. All of these attitudes, assumptions and values are carried over into the physicians' lifelong practice patterns.

How then does palliative care fit into conventional medicine? The World Health Organization defines palliative care as the active total care of the individual where disease is not curable. The goals are the relief of suffering, the control of symptoms and the restoration of functional capacity. These goals are addressed not only through conventional medical approaches but also through psychological, social, cultural and spiritual approaches. The practitioner involved in palliative care is sympathetic to subjective phenomenon such as pain, anxiety, depression and focuses on treating these symptoms directly as important phenomena to address. Similarly, the practitioner is tolerant of incomplete medical knowledge. For example, if the patient has pain, the approaches to treat the pain without necessarily obtaining a CT scan to prove that the metastasis has developed in a particular bony location. Finally and importantly, death is considered as not a defeat but rather the natural conclusion of life. As such, the physician and the entire health care team is devoted to dealing with the patient and the patient's family in a way to ensure comfort.

But it is not only in the setting of an incurable disease where the patient's demise is expected in some fairly definitive time period where this approach to medicine is important. I would propose that science-based medicine, or conventional medicine, needs to shift from the curative model of medical care to a holistic model of medical care. This model is not unlike the model practiced by our forebears just a few generations ago albeit without the benefits of today's scientifically delivered new technologies. It would take today's science-based medicine and add to it symptom-based therapy, attention to preventive medicine, attention to psychosocial needs, and attention to spiritual needs. Thus, the relief of pain, a focus on diet and exercise, attention to stress reduction, and the use of techniques such as massage, will all help to relieve symptoms and to prevent illness in the future. Arranging for financial counseling and developing effective measures of home health care will assist the psychological and family needs of the patient. Teaching the patient meditation will help reduce stress, and being comfortable discussing prayer will help attend to the spiritual needs of the patient. Thus, the purpose of the physician begins to shift from one where cure is the major focus of attention to one where healing becomes the primary focus. The term "healing" implies much more than just cure or care but rather suggests an attention to all of the needs of the patient irrespective of whether an underlying disease can ultimately be cured. It is within this context that I would like to address complementary medicine which I believe can be of assistance in a holistic approach to medicine, one in which the model is that of healing.

Alternative and complementary medicine—definitions, prevalence and techniques

There is no generally accepted definition of alternative, complementary or unconventional medicine. Until recently, the terms tended to connote "unproved," "untested," "quackery," "charlatanism," etc., and organized medicine made strong efforts to not only discourage their use but to actively ban many approaches, to prevent licensing by nonallopathic practitioners, and to bring suit against those who claimed effectiveness for their therapies. Alternative medicine tends to focus on elements of nature, vitalism, observational rather than experimental science and upon spirituality. The term "alternative medicine" is in more common usage than the term "complementary medicine." Alternative medicine is a somewhat unfortunate term, in my opinion, in that it suggests approaches to be used instead of conventional or scienced-based medicine as opposed to the term "complementary" which tends to suggest approaches that are to be used in conjunction with conventional medicine. I therefore prefer the term "complementary medicine."

Complementary Medicine might include diet, exercise, stress reduction methodologies, or techniques commonly used in the Orient, such as acupuncture, acupressure, meditation, herbal medicine, and the like. Many, if not most of these approaches, are unproved by the standard scientific method, are not taught in medical school or residency programs, and, in general, have been on the fringes of orthodox medicine. Complementary approaches, however, have become more and more common, and a number of medical schools (University of Maryland, Stanford) and hospital systems (Sharp in San Diego, Beth Israel in Boston) are developing formal programs. The National Institutes of Health, in part due to congressional pressure, has created the Office of Alternative Medicine (OAM) which has been established to scientifically evaluate some of these processes and procedures [4].

In January, 1993, Eisenberg et al. [5] published an article in the New England Journal of Medicine on the prevalence, costs and patterns of use of unconventional medicine in the United States of America. They noted that the extent and costs of unconventional therapeutic practices were unknown and conducted a national telephone survey during 1991 of 1,539 adults. With a response rate of 67%, they determined that fully one-third (34%) of respondents had utilized at least one of 16 predefined interventions in the past 12 months. Further, one-third of these individuals visited a provider an average 19 times at an average cost per visit of $27.50 during the past year. Interestingly, the highest use was reported by middle aged adults who had relatively more education and higher incomes. There were more visits to alternative medicine practitioners than to primary care physicians, with a ratio of about 4:3 [5].

The 16 unconventional therapies included relaxation techniques (13% usage reported in prior 12 months), chiropractic (10%), massage (7%), imagery (4%), spiritual healing (4%), commercial weight loss program (4%), life style diets (e.g., macrobiotics) (4%), herbal medicine (3%), plus megavitamin therapy (2%), self help groups (2%), energy healing (1%), biofeedback (1%), hypnosis (1%), homeopathy (1%), acupuncture (<1%), and folk remedies (<1%). Not surprisingly, those who saw a provider were especially likely to do so if using acupuncture, chiropractic, hypnosis, and massage therapy.

Some of the most common medical problems for which these therapies were used included back pain, headache, anxiety, and other musculoskeletal dysfunction. Among those who used one or more of these approaches for serious medical conditions, 83% also sought care from a physician.

Nearly one quarter (24%) of those interviewed who reported having cancer had used one or more unconventional approaches. Most commonly utilized were relaxation techniques, chiropractic, and massage.

Most of those who reported using an unconventional therapy did not so report to their medical doctor. Other than reimbursement for chiropractic, biofeedback, and herbal therapists by some insurance carriers, most unconventional medicine was paid entirely out of pocket. The authors extrapolated the survey to the entire United States population to estimate a total annual outlay of $13.7 billion of which $10.3 billion was out of pocket. The authors concluded that use of unconventional therapy was much greater than generally appreciated and, again, noted that most usage went unreported to the individual physician.

The use of alternative, or complementary, approaches in other countries is likewise common and probably higher than most physicians would anticipate. In the United Kingdom, Finland, The Netherlands, Germany and France, the use of alternative medical therapies ranges from 25-75% of the population seeking medical care. In Japan, it is estimated that $1.3 billion is spent annually for Kampo (herbal) remedies. In China, traditional Chinese medicine (the use of herbal therapy, acupuncture, etc.) is more common in many areas of the country than is conventional medicine. Ayurvedic approach to medical care is the dominant medical methodology in India. A Wall Street Journal article on April 14, 1997 reported that spending for alternative medicine, such as chiropractic, acupuncture and reflexology now amounts to $98 billion per year in the USA which was up about 60% since 1989 according to the article [6].

One of the most notable evaluations of complementary medicine is that conducted by Dean Ornish and his colleagues [7,8] into the reversal of coronary artery disease by a combination of stress management, exercise, and diet modification combined with group support sessions. Patients were men and women, middle aged, who had coronary artery disease documented by arteriography and who were then randomly allocated or not to a program that included a low cholesterol (<5 mg/day) low fat (<10% of total energy intake) vegetarian diet with 15% protein and 75% complex carbohydrate augmented with vitamin B12. All patients had to stop smoking and practice stress management techniques for one hour daily which included a meditation technique. They participated in mild to moderate aerobic exercise three hours per week and participated in group support mechanisms. Experimental and control patients had initial and follow-up coronary arteriograms and also had positron emission tomography (PET) before and five years after initiation of risk factor modification. While one cannot determine from this study whether all or only certain of the modifications were critical to the outcome, the patients showed modest but definitive regression of coronary artery stenosis and decreased size and severity of perfusion abnormalities on rest-dipyridimole PET images. While this work has been published in the *Journal of the American Medical Association* by Gould, et al. [7], it is also recorded in greater detail in a book by Dr. Ornish entitled "Program for Reversing Heart Disease" [9].

Complementary, alternative, and unorthodox medical practices have become common topics for lay publications. Anyone standing in line at the local supermarket will be bombarded with articles in magazines such as *Natural Health, Prevention, Ladies Home Journal*, etc. *Life Magazine* had a major article on alternative medicine during the summer of 1996, and *Consumers Report* had a three-part series entitled "Alternative Medicine: The Facts" in the January, 1994 issue [10].

Why do individuals seek out complementary medicine? A number of studies give some indications. Different attitudes on health and illness appear important. Those seeking complementary medicine in a study of 202 adult working Germans [11] suggest that they were more critical and skeptical as to the effectiveness of orthodox medicine but were not necessarily personally disappointed with the lack of effectiveness in a first-hand manner from their physician. Rather, they simply carried a deep-seated belief that complementary medicine should/will work for them. In a British study of 250 individuals who used acupuncture, homeopathy or osteopathy, the key reasons for using complementary medicine were: "I value the emphasis on treating the whole person," "Because of believe complementary medicine will be more effective than orthodox medicine," "Because I believe complementary medicine will allow me to take a more active part in maintaining my health" [12].

Framework for use of complementary medicine

In focusing on complementary medicine for the palliative care of patients with cancer or AIDS, I would suggest that the concepts enunciated by Lerner [13] form a sound framework. He begins by noting the distinction between healing and curing akin to the concept of the medical model of holistic, or healing, care described at the beginning of this chapter. Lerner notes that healing may be physical, mental or spiritual or any combination of the three. Healing enhances the quality of life and it may or may not lengthen the span of life. Importantly, healing is in the domain of the patient not the physician. The patient is the one in charge and the physician and other health care providers are in the service of the patient.

Using these concepts, it follows that conventional medicine should be the primary approaches to the treatment of cancer or AIDS. In all likelihood, there are no complementary approaches which are curative. On the other hand, complementary approaches may well assist in the supportive care of the patient and equally, if not more importantly, complementary approaches may help in healing.

The uses of complementary medicine in cancer or AIDS should be considered from the following perspective. First, complementary medicine techniques are not curative, and there is little scientific evidence for their effect on symptomatic relief. On the other hand, there is strong antidotal evidence for improved quality of life. It is notable that the average user is above average in education, income and in motivation, and the average practitioner is both licensed and charges fees [13].

In searching for choices in healing, Lerner focuses on five approaches (Table 1). Spiritual approaches including prayer and hands-on approaches; psychological approaches would include support groups and guided imagery or creative visualization; nutritional approaches including diet and other supplements; and physical approaches would include massage, yoga and perhaps chiropractic. Lerner believes that these four approaches represent a "vital quartet" he believes may enhance the quality of life and improve functional status for patients with cancer. He adds a fifth approach which is the use of traditional medical systems such as Chinese (including acupuncture and herbal therapy), Ayurvedic medicine which uses mental and emotional approaches plus a variety of herbal compounds, traditional European herbal medicines and traditional Native American approaches. The Chinese, India Ayurvedic, and Native American Indian approaches have long empirical traditions, and European herbal remedies were well known and followed by Americans from colonial times until just a generation or two ago.

Table 1. Choices in healing [13]

Spiritual: prayer, hands-on*
Psychological: support groups, imagery*
Nutritional: diet, supplements*
Physical: massage, yoga, chiropractic*
Traditional Medicine: Chinese, Ayurvedic**

---

* "Vital Quartet" – May enhance quality of life and improve functional status; ** Long empirical traditions

SPECIFIC COMPLEMENTARY MEDICINE APPROACHES TO SUPPORTIVE CARE OF CANCER AND AIDS

Acupuncture

Acupuncture has been shown to be an effective adjunct to reduce emesis after chemotherapy. Vickers [14] reviewed 33 controlled trials in the literature from which he selected 12 as being of particularly high quality as both randomized and placebo-controlled. In each of these investigations, the P6 acupuncture site was utilized. In 11 of the 12 trials with over 2,000 patients studied, acupuncture proved to be statistically superior to placebo.

Acupuncture needles can be inserted and left alone, can be twirled, or can be attached through minor electric current. A related approach is transcutaneous electrical nerve stimulation (TENS) which has been found useful for pain control. Acupuncture, electroacupuncture and TENS have all been found to be useful in reducing chemotherapy-induced nausea and vomiting. In an Irish study involving 130 patients with repeated episodes of chemotherapy-induced emesis, electroacupuncture was either completely or considerably effective in 97% of patients. Sham acupuncture sites, even though electrically stimulated, do not have the beneficial effects. Unfortunately, the effect is relatively short-lived. TENS was then studied by the same investigators [15], and they found that in over 100 patients with chemotherapy-induced emesis, 75% had considerable benefit. Although less than electroacupuncture, the benefit of TENS was that it could be self-administered by patients every two hours for a longer lasting relief [15].

There is substantial data on the use of acupuncture for pain relief [16]. Some studies at the University of Maryland School of Medicine are illustrative of the use of acupuncture for musculoskeletal pain. Brian M. Berman, M.D. was recruited to establish a complementary medicine program in 1991. Starting with a $1 million grant from the Maurice Laing Foundation and Thera Trust in London, Berman has set out to establish a scientific basis for a number of complementary medical procedures, such as acupuncture. In this regard, he and his colleagues have now shown in pilot controlled trials that patients with severe osteoarthritis of the knee receiving best medical therapy will have decreased need for pain medication and increased mobility through the added use of acupuncture. This was a double-blinded trial in which Berman gave real or sham acupuncture to patients who then recorded their use of pain medication while their rheumatologist recorded range of motion [17]. In another study, individuals having their wisdom teeth removed were or were not given acupuncture [18]. Those who received acupuncture treatments reported less pain following the procedure, used less pain medications, and used them for a shorter period of time. In an animal model, Berman and colleagues have demonstrated that acupuncture releases endorphins into the cerebrospinal fluid suggesting at least one aspect of the physiology of the potential physiological effect of acupuncture.

Mind-body techniques

Meditation/relaxation response

Mind-body techniques have been described in a multipart network television series moderated by Bill Moyers and subsequently published as a best seller [19]. A commonly utilized mind-body technique is meditation which has been shown to reduce blood pressure, induce a sense of well being and reduce both anxiety and depression [20,21]. One of the earliest to scientifically study mind-body approaches was Herbert Benson, M.D., a cardiologist originally of Harvard and later of Tufts Medical School, who popularized what he calls the "relaxation response" [22]. He had been studying approaches to hypertension when he met some individuals from India who said that they could teach him meditation techniques which would lower blood pressure. Initially skeptical, he began to study meditation and determined that, indeed, it did reduce blood pressure and change pulse rate in addition to creating a general calming effect and inducing a sense of increased energy. In developing his methodology with patients, he chose to avoid the term "meditation" because of its sometimes "exotic" connotations and instead coined the term "relaxation response." This is a fairly simplified form of meditation in which the patient is asked to focus on a single word or short phrase. The word can have some religious connotation to the individual, such as "Lord," or it can be a word with little or no other meaning, such as "one." The purpose, however, is to quiet the mind and focus it on this one word so as to prevent the wandering or "chattering" that occurs within the conscious brain all of the time. Individuals who practice this technique have been regularly shown to reduce their blood pressure and/or reduce or eliminate their need for antihypertensive medications, especially when done in concert with diet and exercise [22].

Hatha yoga

Hatha yoga, a technique of simple, quiet stretching exercises with a quiet peaceful attitude, tones the musculature, creates a serene, quiet mind and is often employed as an adjunct or as a precursor to meditation [9,23].

Visualization/guided imagery

Visualization and guided imagery are related mind-body techniques. With creative visualization, an individual seeks a quiet resting state in a semi-meditative mode in which they imagine themselves as healthy, free of disease, free of certain habits such as smoking, overeating, or enthused about positive attributes such as exercise. The concept is that if one repetitively embeds a desired state into the subconscious mind, the mind-body connections will work toward that state in an ongoing fashion. Guided imagery is a similar technique in which the patient imagines elements of the body actively affecting a disease; e.g., macrophages and natural killer cells are imagined as moving toward the tumor and destroying it.

Support groups

There are now over 45 studies which demonstrate that support groups, or psychosocial interventions, will enhance the quality of life [24]. It is important to recall that the cancer or AIDS patients' major concerns are the fear of dying alone (be this literally or figuratively) and of unmanaged pain. These are not necessarily the physicians' primary concerns in dealing with the patient. In support groups, the concept is to help the patient learn how to cope better so that they can have improved interaction with physicians and other medical team members; so that they can manage pain on their own to a greater degree through relaxation techniques and self-hypnosis; through teaching various relaxation skills such as meditation or deep breathing; and in teaching the patient problem-solving skills. The group setting is generally conducive to these approaches, in part, because patients can gain from one another and recognize that they are not alone in their concerns, anxieties and frustrations. As a generalization, the studies of support groups have demonstrated that overall quality of life is much improved; that the patients have better pain management and coping skills; that there is less psychological distress, including reduced anxiety and reduced depression; and there is increased physical activity. It may be worth noting that complementary medicine practitioners typically spend more time with their patients; more time addressing symptoms as opposed to the underlying disease; and more time focusing on the patient's concerns. Thus, complementary medicine practitioners are much more likely to be involved with support group type activities in a direct or indirect way than are physicians.

There are within these 45 evaluations three studies with a total of 250 patients who have demonstrated longer survival or reduced mortality rates as a result of psychosocial interventions [24]. One of these studies, by David Spiegel and associates at Stanford has been commonly referred to since its publication in *The Lancet* in 1989. Eighty-six women with metastatic breast cancer were randomly allocated to psychosocial interventions (50) or not (36). All patients had standard oncologic care whereas those randomized to intervention had weekly supportive group therapy that lasted for 90 minutes and were trained in self-hypnosis for pain. It is to be noted that the study was prospective but was not designed to study survival but rather to address psychological distress and pain management. Thus, the authors did not control for potential survival factors so that there was no attempt to balance, for example, the disease stages other than that all women had metastases. At the end of the first year, the results demonstrated that there was decreased anxiety and decreased pain among the patients. At follow-up ten years later at which time only three of the patients were still alive, there was a clear difference in survival. The control patients had lived an average of 19 months whereas the support group patients had lived an average of 37 months, a statistically significant difference. When analyzed with a Kaplan-Meier survival plot, it was demonstrated that a divergence of survival began at 20 months after randomization (or eight months after intervention ended), again statistically significant [25].

In another study, Fawzy, et al. at UCLA School of Medicine evaluated the recurrence of survival of 68 patients with malignant melanoma who participated in a six week structured psychiatric group intervention which took place shortly after their diagnosis and initial surgical treatment. The groups were then observed for about six years. Patients were randomly allocated to either no intervention or intervention which consisted of teaching of a psychosocial intervention which, among other things, taught coping skills, relaxation, pain management skills, and problem-solving skills. They found that these interventions enhanced effective coping and reduced affective distress and, in addition, found that there were more deaths (10 of 34) among the control patients than in the intervention patients (3 of 34), a statistically significant difference [26]. A third study by Richardson shows a survival advantage as a result of a supportive educational program among patients with leukemias and lymphomas. In this latter study, the supportive program was relatively brief and was actually designed to enhance medical compliance unlike the other studies where there was a more defined approach to psychosocial intervention. They found an increase in social support, self-care and sense of control by the patients in addition to a survival advantage [27]. These are relatively small studies and generally were not designed to address survival; nontheless, they are intriguing. In any event, they each demonstrate improved quality of life.

Prayer

Finally, prayer is a form of complementary medicine that needs to be considered as part of mind/body techniques. Larry Dossey, M.D., editor of Alternative Therapies, A Journal of Alternative Medicine, has written a "best seller" which focuses, in part, on prayer as an adjunct to medical care [28]. One scientific evaluation of prayer therapy was done at San Francisco General Hospital. Cardiologist Randolph Byrd of UCSF, conducted a 10 month study in which 393 patients admitted to the coronary care unit were randomly allocated to either be in a group that was prayed for by home prayer groups or to a group that was not remembered in prayer. It was a randomized, prospectively, double blind trial. The prayer givers were individuals recruited for this purpose with no personal knowledge of the patients and with no specific instructions as to how they should pray other than to do so at least once each day. Prayer groups were given the names of patients; each patient had five to seven people praying for him or her. The prayed-for patients were five times less likely than the unremembered patients to require antibiotics (3 versus 16 patients); they were less likely to develop pulmonary edema (6 versus 18); less likely to require endotracheal intubation (0 versus 12 patients); and fewer prayed-for patients died, although the difference was not statistically significant [29].

Tying mind-body medicine together as a scientific discipline is the concept of psychoneuroimmunology, or the study of CNS function on physiologic processes. This area has grown rapidly in the past 10-15 years as evidenced by a symposium entitled "Psychoneuroimmunology and cancer: fifteenth Sapporo cancer seminar [30]. The report of the symposium in *Cancer Research* gives a good overview of the interactions, as currently understood, between the brain and the endocrine/immune systems.

Massage

The word "massage" comes from Arabic meaning "to stroke." There are records of massage having been used in China at least 3,000 years ago and in Egypt 4,200 years ago. Hippocrates was a very strong advocate of the use of massage, and it was a common form of medical therapy in Europe until the Middle Ages when the Catholic church denounced it as "the work of the Devil." More recently, the association of massage with prostitution has given it a bad reputation, but the increasing emphasis on healthy lifestyles has brought massage back in the United States to a position of relatively common acceptance. For example, some companies now employ massage therapists as a employee benefit to reduce stress and increase relaxation while on the job.

In some medical studies of massage, it has been well demonstrated that premature infants who receive massage compared to those who are not massaged are more alert, active and responsive; they gain weight nearly 50% faster; they sleep more deeply, their hospital stay is about six days shorter, and the total cost is about $10,000 less. Despite this, the use of massage for premature infants has not become a covered expense and is rarely a standard therapeutic practice [31].

Massage has been shown to lead to improvement for some patients with asthma; it has been demonstrated to cause some increase in immune function in HIV infected patients; it increases concentration in autistic children; it substantially lessens anxiety in burn victims about to undergo debridement; it lessens depression and reduces frequency of migraine headaches [31].

Interestingly, there is some controversy as to whether some patients with cancer should undergo massage. Those who are opposed suggest that it might increase circulation to areas of cancer and, hence, increase tumor growth or that it might promote metastases. On the other side are those who give and those who receive massage who report profound relaxation, reduction of chronic pain and reduction of tension. In addition, the psychological benefit of the hands-on effect of massage can be very positive. Kay Warren in *Nursing Times* [32] recommends low stroke back massage along with distraction, guided imagery and progressive muscle relaxation to enhance relaxation and the general feeling of well being among patients with cancer. Also in *Nursing Times* [33], S. Sims, in a pilot study, reported that breast cancer patients had fewer symptoms, had more tranquility and more vitality with less tension and tiredness as a result of massage therapy.

Massage by a massage therapist is well known to have stress reducing benefits which can be of value to a cancer patient without having any direct effect on the cancer per se. Other approaches are modern offshoots of the ancient concept of "laying on of hands." The concept is that there is an energy field which exists around each person, and that this energy field can be altered through the efforts of a practitioner. These types of approaches have become fairly popular in the United States in recent years.

Other touch therapies

The concept of "laying on of hands" goes back into the far reaches of history. One technique used today and known as "Therapeutic Touch" had been developed from this background largely by Dora Kunz, a healer, and Delores Krieger, a professor of nursing at New York University [34]. Krieger teaches the concept and believes that essentially anyone can learn the technique, Therapeutic Touch. The approach includes three phases. In the first phase, centering, the healer enters a meditative state to become acutely open to any input from the client. In the second phase, assessing, the therapist scans a patient's body with hands held a few inches above the skin to detect disturbances in the energy field around the body. The third phase, rebalancing, uses the therapist's hands to smooth out the energy field. The procedure takes about 15-20 minutes. Therapeutic Touch has been taught to nurses across the country and is used at multiple institutions, hospices and in offices. In research studies, Therapeutic Touch seems to be effective in reducing acute pain in postoperative patients, in relieving pain in general, decreasing anxiety in hospitalized patients, improving behavior in premature infants and decreasing headache pain in adults.

COMMENTS

Ornish's studies of cardiac disease used multiple interventions at once: diet, smoking cessation, exercise, relaxation techniques, meditation, hatha yoga and group support. While it is impossible to dissect out which elements were or were not critical to the improved outcome, the results were clear: a demonstrable reduction in coronary artery narrowing and improved cardiac muscle perfusion. Perhaps with cancer or AIDS patients, the same approach can be considered. Physicians should consider use of those techniques that seem to add benefit to the patient's symptoms and improve the quality of life. Concurrently, we need to await the outcome of scientific studies of each modality.

Complementary medicine has a clear role in palliative care of cancer and AIDS. If one is to follow a holistic approach to medical care, one in which the focus is on healing and not just an attempt at cure of the underlying disease, then complementary medicine techniques are clearly appropriate. True, they have not received the type of scientific validation that might be desirable, but to the extent that the patient finds relief and has an improved quality of life as a result of these techniques, then the use of complementary techniques is clearly valid and appropriate. Furthermore, it is clear that patients use complementary approaches with or without their doctor's knowledge or recommendation, and it therefore behooves physicians to recognize that their patients may well be visiting complementary medical practitioners. That being the case, it is better that physician and complementary medicine practitioner work together as a team, understanding what each team member can add to the overall care and healing of the patient [35]. Acupuncture, electroacupuncture and transcutaneous nerve stimulation can all be used to reduce chemotherapy-induced nausea and emesis, they can reduce pain, and they can be useful for other syndromes such as migraines. Herbal remedies have been used for thousands of years and some seem to be useful in reducing stress, a calming influence, perhaps reducing the side effects of chemotherapy, as a "tonic," and just the general pleasant effects of a good cup of tea. The mind-body approaches of meditation can reduce stress or create a positive mental attitude. Massage can reduce stress, reduce pain and, in general, energize the recipient. These practices need to be incorporated into the curriculum of academic medical centers so that the physicians know and understand these techniques, but, more importantly, is the need for a fundamental shift from the curative model to the holistic model of medical care which focuses on the patient and not the disease. The holistic medical model will recognize that the cure of disease is not the only goal of medicine; recognize that its symptoms are worthy of direct treatment; accept death as the natural conclusion of life when the underlying disease cannot be cured; and accept that true holistic medicine includes attention to psychological, social, cultural and spiritual concerns and needs of the patient and the patient's family. Once the holistic model of medical care is accepted, complementary approaches will become part of the mainstream.

REFERENCES

1. Fox E (1997) Predominance of the curative model of medical care. A residual problem. JAMA 278: 761-763
2. Billings JA, Block S (1997) Palliative care in undergraduate medical education. Status report and future directions. JAMA 278: 733-738
3. Christakis DA, Feudtner C (1997) Temporary matters: the ethical consequences of transient social relationships in medical training. JAMA 278: 739-743
4. Gordon JS (1996) Alternative medicine and the family physician. Am Family Phys 54: 2205-2210
5. Eisenberg DM, Kessler RC, Foster C, Norlock FE, Calkins DR, Delbanco TL (1993) Unconventional medicine in the United States. N Engl J Med 328: 246-252
6. Wall Street Journal, April 14, 1997, p B1
7. Gould KL, Ornish D, Scherwitz L, Brown S, Edens RP, Hess MJ, Mullani N, Bolomey L, Dobbs F, Armstrong WT, Merritt T, Ports T, Sparler S, Billings J (1995) Changes in myocardial perfusion abnormalities by positron emission tomography after long-term, intense risk factor modification. JAMA 274: 894-901
8. Ornish D, Brown SB, Scherwitz LW, Billings JH, Armstrong WT, Ports TA, et al. (1990) Can life style changes reverse coronary heart disease? The Lifestyle Heart Trial. Lancet 336: 129-133
9. Ornish D (1990) Program for reversing heart disease. Ballantine Books, New York
10. Alternative medicine: the facts (1994) Consumer's Report, January
11. Furnham A, Kirkcaldy B (1996) The health beliefs and behaviors of orthodox and complementary medicine clients. Br J Clin Psychol 35: 49-61
12. Vincent C, Furnham A (1996) Why do patients turn to complementary medicine? An empirical study. Br J Clin Psychol 35: 37-48
13. Lerner M (1994) Choices in healing: integrating the best of conventional and complementary approaches to cancer. MIT Press, Cambridge, MA

14. Vickers AJ (1996) Can acupuncture have specific effects on health? A systematic review of acupuncture antiemesis trials. J R Soc Med 89: 303-311

15. Dundee JW (1990) Belfast experience with P6 acupunture antiemesis. Ulster Med J 59: 63-70

16. Thomas M (1997) Acupuncture studies on patient. Acupunc Med 15: 23-31

17. Berman BM, Lao L, Greene M, Anderson RW, Wong RH, Langenberg P, Hochberg M (1995) Efficacy of traditional Chinese acupuncture in the treatment of symptomatic knee osteoarthritis: a pilot study. Osteoarth Cartil 3: 139-142

18. Lao L, Wong RL, Berman BM (1995) Efficacy of Chinese acupuncture on post operative oral surgery pain. Oral Surg Oral Med Oral Pathol 79: 423-428

19. Moyers B (1993) Healing and the mind. Doubleday, New York

20. Cooper M, Aygen M (1978) Effect of meditation on blood cholesterol and blood pressure. Harefuah 95: 1-2

21. Chopra D (1989) Quantum healing: Exploring the frontiers of mind-body medicine. Bantam Books, New York

22. Benson H (1975) The relaxation response. William Morrow, New York

23. Gore MM (1982) Effect of yogic treatment on some pulmonary functions in asthmatics. Yoga Mimamsa 20: 51-58

24. Dreher H (1997) The scientific and moral imperative for broad-based psychosocial interventions for cancer. Advances: J Mind-Body Health 13: 38-49

25. Spiegel D, Bloom J, Kraemer HC et al. (1989) Effect of psychosocial treatment on survival of patients with metastatic breast cancer. Lancet 2: 888-891

26. Fawzy FI, Fawzy NW, Hyun CS, Elashoff R, Guthrie D, Fahey JL, Morton DL (1993) Malignant melanoma: effects of an early structured psychiatric intervention, coping, and affective state on recurrence and survival 6 years later. Arch Gen Psychiatry 50: 681-689

27. Richardson JL, Shelton DR, Krailo M, Levine AM (1990) The effect of compliance with treatment on survival among patients with hematologic malignancies. J Clin Oncol 8: 356-364

28. Dossey L (1989) Recovering the soul: a scientific and spiritual search. Bantam Books, New York

29. Byrd RC (1988) Positive therapeutic effects of intercessory prayer in a coronary care unit population. South Med J 81: 826-829

30. Besedovsky HO, Herberman RB, Temoshok LR, Sendo F (1996) Psychoneuro-immunology and cancer: fifteenth Sapporo cancer seminar meeting report. Cancer Res 56: 4278-4281

31. Field T (1995) Massage therapy for infants and children. J Develop Behav Ped 16: 105-111

32. Warren K (1988) "Will I be sick, nurse?" Nurs Times 84: 53-54

33. Sims S (1986) Slow stroke back massage for cancer patients. Nurs Times 82: 47-50

34. Krieger D (1975) Therapeutic touch: the imprimatur of nursing. Am J Nurs 75: 784-787

35. Eisenberg DM (1997) Advising patients who seek alternative medical therapies. Ann Intern Med 127: 61-69

SUPPORT WITH INFORMATION, EDUCATION AND COUNSELLING IN PATIENTS WITH ADVANCED CANCER AND AIDS

Mayumi ABE, RGN
Bank Nurse, St Christopher's Hospice, London, UK

SUMMARY. People are increasingly being encouraged to accept responsibility for their own health, well-being and for their future. Health professionals have recognised this and the willingness of many patients to participate in their care. We should respond and try to develop new models of practice and flexibility of attitude to cater for individual needs.

Patients with life-threatening illnesses are living longer and getting more and more complex treatment so the health professionals need to become more expert in helping to cope with both the illness and its treatment.

The quality of life becomes more important than the quantity.

I personally am very interested in the support, education and counselling needs of patients with AIDS and cancer, from early stages of diagnosis, during active treatment and hopefully palliative care in the different states of their disease. During these times patients' needs are continually changing so we need to be adaptable.

Since I have been in England, I have seen a different kind of nursing and have begun to take an interest in the quality of nursing for advanced cancer patients and HIV/AIDS patients.

This paper examines how effective is the care given to patients with life-threatening illnesses from my experience as a nurse, and looking back, how it affected me as well. It also examines a better understanding of human behaviour in life-threatening illnesses.

KEYWORDS: Palliative Care, Support, Counselling, Communication

INTRODUCTION

The reason I have become interested in palliative care was because many questions came to my mind following an incident with a patient I was looking after when working as a volunteer at the London Hospital. For the sake of the story I will call her Mary and she was a lady in her late 40's suffering from cancer. When I met her for the first time she openly said to me:

> "I know I have cancer. As far as I'm concerned I'm glad. I know what I have... Life is not forever. I found that the doctors and nurses were very supportive to me. I'm going to die tomorrow!" And she did.

As I was so surprised at her talking like this, I spoke to someone in the hospital. She was a clinical specialist nurse in palliative care who had been aware of Mary's situation and had gained her trust. She said that Mary had been told her diagnosis and had had time to come to terms with her illness and wanted to make the most of the time she had left. The encounter with Mary highlighted the importance to me of palliative care which provides both physical and psychological support from the time of diagnosis through to the terminal stage of illness.

This made me think of how things were back home in Japan and how we care for patients with life-threatening illness. Mary's attitude helped towards changing my views, as in the past I have seen many patients go through much anguish because they wanted to know their diagnosis but no one would tell them.

So my questions were "should patients be told the truth? Does the patient actually realise that they don't have long to live? How does the care of a patient with a terminal illness differ from other areas of health care?"

To find the answers to these questions and many others I decided to study palliative care which has developed from caring for dying patients and established itself in the Hospice Movement started by Dr Cicely Saunders and this is where I have since worked and studied.

So my experience was seen as a great asset. I felt comfortable and confident in the presence of the fear and misery of patients with cancer and AIDS. There has been a heightened interest in these people's needs, to try to sensitively understand and enhance the quality of care. I hope to make my contribution to good practice in life-threatening illness to care in the hospital or hospice or community.

The most common response is for the health professional to try to impose their own views, for want of anything "better to do". So in each case the question needs to be asked about the value of human life. This needs to be expanded into a question about the nature of human life, here and now.

What is palliative care?

Palliative care is defined as:

> The active total care of patients whose disease is not responsive to curative treatment. Control of pain, of other symptoms, and of psychological, social and spiritual problems is paramount. The goal of palliative care is achievement of the best quality of life for patients and their families.
>
> WHO 1990 (1)

The Department of Health, in the Calman-Hine Report, defined palliative care as:

> Palliative care should not be associated exclusively with terminal care. Many patients need it early in the course of their disease, sometimes from the time of diagnosis. The palliative care team should integrate in a seamless way with all cancer treatment services to provide the best possible quality of life for the patient and their family.
>
> (2)

Higginson expands on this definition, commenting that the term was originally used only for terminally ill people "but it is now broadened to include the care of those who have a life-threatening disease but are not imminently dying, including people who have recently been diagnosed with cancer and those who have other life-threatening diseases such as multiple sclerosis, motor neurone disease, AIDS or chronic circulatory or respiratory disease."

(3)

The Palliative Care Approach

The palliative care approach aims to present both physical and psychological well-being and is an integral part of all clinical practice, whatever the illness or its stage, from the point of diagnosis when appropriate. The key principles underpinning palliative care comprise:

Whole person approach

Care which encompassed both the patient and those who matter to them

Emphasis on open and sensitive communication, including adequate information about diagnosis and treatment options

Respect for patient autonomy and choice

Focus on quality of life which includes good symptom control.

(4)

Development of Palliative Care Services

Palliative care is a recent but rapidly expanding field. It is generally recognised to have developed during the 1960's from the pioneering work of Dame Cicely Saunders in the UK.
In the UK hospice and specialist palliative services have expanded rapidly during the last 30 years.

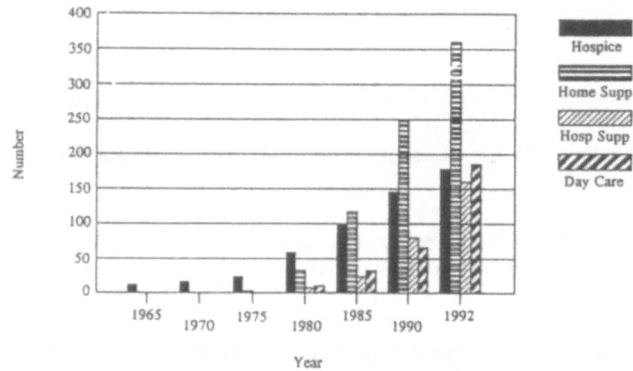

Growth in hospices, support teams and day care between 1967 and 1992
in the UK and Republic of Ireland.

Higginson, I 1993   (3)

Why is it still so difficult to provide the Information?

The one clear fact is that there is no easy answer to the problem to tell or not to tell. Often for the patient cancer or AIDS is simply another word for a painful death.

Sontag (1991) has pointed out, illness as a figure where there are many different taboos and misconceptions regarding such as cancer and AIDS. Among both professionals and the general public, fear of the disease is a dominant theme. This is something we have to deal with. AIDS is often a secret, but not from the patient. We need to learn to regard cancer as if it were just a disease - a very serious one, but just a disease, not a curse, not a punishment, not an embarrassment.

Without meaning and not necessarily a death sentence.

(5)

The social impact of cancer and AIDS as related partly to community lack of understanding and the health professionals' lack of confidence and lack of knowledge generally go hand in hand with poor quality of care for the life-threatening illness.

Webb P points out:

> "Perhaps the most significant socio-cultural issue influencing patient information provision is that of paternalism". The problem of paternalism is not only between health professionals and patients, but often a problem between patients and their relatives or frients and usually stems from a desire to protect the patient."

(6)

Most patients have a pretty accurate idea of the general nature of their illness. Most of them have already sensed it. This is an inevitable source of distress, in life-threatening illness, for we are afraid of uncertainty, negative feelings, loss of control and threat of loss of self-esteem.

> "He fears the unknown more than the known.
> He fears professional disinterest more than professional ineptitude.
> He fears the process of dying more than death itself.
> He fears isolation, whether physical or psychological"

(7)

Uncertainty is a stressful factor as the individual wonders "What is wrong with me?"

There are undoubtedly some patients who do not wish to face the truth and who will continue to push it out of their minds.

> It is important for health professionals to remember that some people prefer not to know too much, while others demand to know everything.

(8)

It is, I believe, our moral, legal and professional duty to help the patient reach this understanding, so that he/she has a clear idea of the options available, and is able to give his/her consent to treatment and investigation.

How to Break Bad News

Information about their treatment, options, the likelihood of treatment success and possible side-effects were considered particularly important. The information need of patients varied from person to person and changed as they progressed through diagnosis, treatment and follow-up. The information provided should, therefore, be relevant to this particular phase of the life-threatening illness journey and to the individual.

Regarding telling the truth - the information does belong to the patient, so we must respect people's autonomy, assist their preparation to cope by providing support and we must respond to their life.

Buckman's Breaking Bad News - a six-step practical

Step 1 Getting started: who should be there?

Step 2 Finding out how much the patient knows

Step 3 Finding out how much the patient wants to know

Step 4 Sharing the information (aligning and educating)
      (diagnosis - treatment: plan - prognosis - support)

Step 5 Responding to the patient's feelings

Step 6 Planning and follow-through

---

(9)

Patients' information needs varied - not all wanted to know everything and very few wanted to know everything at once, but most patients wanted to be able to ask, knowing they would receive an honest answer and that they could keep on asking until they felt that their particular need for information had been satisfied. Patients felt that information should be a two-way process and that health professionals needed information about their patients if they were to be effective.

(10)

The diagnosis of life-threatening illness and psychological reaction of every patient is different, but certain common patterns recur.

Acute distress as the full reality dawns, anxiety, anger, denial, guilt, bargaining and protest, often lasting several weeks.

Depression and despair, which may also last several weeks.

Gradual adjustment and acceptance, often taking several months.

We need to create a critical mass of health professionals who are skilled at helping individuals and understanding their feelings and thoughts through counselling and support.

Coping with the Life-Threatening Illness Experience

For a person diagnosed with life-threatening illness such as cancer, AIDS and their families it is this awareness which happens during a very traumatic and emotional time of their lives. They need especially someone who is willing to be there, to share all their fears, anxieties, hopes, anger, not to judge or criticise, just be there. I feel that it is vital to remember that each patient and each family member is an individual with ideals and ideas which are very individual and unique to him or her.

However, in supporting the individual's growth toward a new awareness of 'being' through the living life, the health professional has a very important duty in communicating with the patient and family, and can assess how best to convey information to them. Everyone is different and the ways people handle information can differ greatly.

One issue involves the right to be told that they have cancer. To what extent should options available to the patient be explained, so that the patient is involved in the choices made about the future? We also need to be aware that information belongs to the patients, as do their bodies and also their future. The truth can actually be a relief for the patients and carers in sharing the burden.

Education need

Education for cancer and AIDS patient need is to improve physical and psychological well-being and enable the patients to cope more effectively with living with their illness.

Patients seeking an understanding of events throughout the course of their journey. Health professionals must recognise their limitations.

Gran (1996) identified eleven types of "elements of an effective patient education program" need.

(11)

1.   Awareness of information as a fundamental human right.

2.   The right of self-determination.

3.   The value of fair distribution of power.

4.   Honesty, as to truth-telling.

5.   The importance of interaction.

6.   Understanding as a care concept.

7.   Structure to avoid conflicting messages.

8.   Learning needs assessment.

9.   Appropriateness for the adult learner.

10.   Involving the patient's partner.

11.   Availability of information at the 'right' time.

I think knowledge is vital in order to be supportive along with honesty and sincerity, these will help to prove the person is not 'on their own'.

Counselling Need

The sharing of information with patients through active listening and being present with the individual, providing encouragement for them to express feelings, giving support and guidance to them.

Counselling, emotional support and practical activity by health professionals permit the understanding of the total situation of the whole person and their family.

Counselling gives a person the opportunity to discover, explore and clarify ways of living more resourcefully and towards greater well-being. (British Association of Counselling 1978). Emotional difficulties as a result of life-threatening illness are not always easy to talk about and are often hardest to share with others. We need to provide counselling skills to help people talk about their thoughts, feelings and ideas. Some patients may be able to express themselves freely, whereas others deny symptoms or reject the nature of their illness.

It is important that a professional gives the patient permission to be him- or herself, is non-judgemental, and understands these responses.

So the expression of need is unique to each individual. The whole range of a person's life experiences influences the nature and uniqueness of that person's spirituality, shaping a unique capacity to respond to all life's events and situations.

Support Need

Since I have been in the UK I found it is the same for many patients with life-threatening illnesses in that they have a need for openness and trust in the patient-health care professional relationship. The health professional must be sympathetic, be a good listener, be open and understanding, be available and explore the medical problems clearly, be flexible about therapeutic options and second options. There must also be time, time to discuss fears and explain future plans, time and opportunity to decide and choose which treatment should be asked for, time to be treated as a person.

Professionals should focus support for the patient and family from the time of diagnosis of the disease. What we should be doing is offering support.

However, in order to achieve a meaningful relationship in which they can gain emotional comfort and support, honesty must prevail.

Health professionals can also encourage the patient to live a normal and independent existence, maintaining self-esteem and dignity by treating the patient as an individual and providing the knowledge and opportunity to make decisions and maintain control of his or her life. We have to realise that without good relationships with patients it is impossible for patients to build a working relationship with health professionals. Sensitivity, approachability and willingness to listen and explain, respect and honesty were considered essential attributes for health professionals caring for those with life-threatening illnesses.

Firstly, to relieve pain and other distressing symptoms. We have to develop a philosophy of dealing with these patients and their families. The World Health Organisation analysis ladder for treating cancer pain has been proven effective in a high percentage of patients. Physical pain is often caused anxiety, fear, worries. Whereas pain must be considered a key component of the quality of life, other symptoms become of greater importance when pain is controlled. The quality of the brief time remaining for the patient is likely to be more important than its length.

Secondly, to create an environment of security. Nevertheless, communication between patients and health professionals is vitally important and should aim to convey to the patient a feeling of security and trust. An understanding of the disease, practical and decision making more effectively that seeking information is an important coping strategy for the patient early in the disease process.

Thirdly, to give emotional, social and spiritual support for patients, to help them come to terms with their own anger, disappointment, depression, resentment and sometimes withdrawal which prevents them communicating meaningfully with patients. Nurses have time to talk and listen to patients and to help them come to terms with their psychological problems relating to the life-threatening illness. It is vital in order to effectively support people during this traumatic time of their lives. If patients are referred at the beginning of their illness, it gives the patient and the nurse time to build up a support and hopefully the last stages of their disease will be less stressful as problems can be talked through as they occur and not left until the last few days of life. Recognition of individual coping styles - human beings face death in different ways.

Fourthly, to help the patient enjoy their remaining life to the full, helping to make family decisions, repair old rifts with friends and most of all achieve peace of a mental and spiritual kind. The patient will be comfortable and have peace of mind, and remain in control of his or her life. It is not necessary to keep him or her in the hospital - he or she may be far happier living a normal life at home. At least this is his or her familiar world and security. Warn the family how difficult it will be, but that the responsibility for the patients' happiness is theirs and best provided at home on a day-to-day basis.

Fifthly, the family play an important part of the care of cancer patients and AIDS patients. The whole situation is extremely devastating and stressful and the nurse can make it easier to cope by giving adequate information, getting to know the relatives, offering support, advice and, if appropriate, encouraging the relatives to feel worthwhile, they cope better if they feel that they are doing something and this will help them through their grief.

Finally, in the UK there are numerous sources of information and groups available for patients with cancer and AIDS and their families and relatives. For example, BACUP, CancerLink, Macmillan Cancer Relief Fund, National AIDS Helpline, and these provide help by telephone, and publish information leaflets.

Case History 1

I am going to close by presenting two case histories, the first is about M., a widow in her 40's, who was a political refugee from Uganda, arrived in the UK in 1991, after her husband had been murdered by the regime in power. She had three sons who remained in Uganda, aged 20, 15 and 13. She lived alone here. When she heard she was HIV positive she was very shocked and said that she hadn't had a boyfriend and didn't know anyone with 'disease' and 'Uganda doesn't have a problem with this disease'. She denied being HIV positive until shortly before her death. She then accepted the truth. She knew she had AIDS though she did use the word shock by diagnosis. When she became unable to manage to stay at home she agreed to accept a visit from the District Nurse and the hospice home care nurse.

She was admitted to a hospice for symptom control. During her stay in the hospice she was extremely angry. She was angry at her complete loss of control and at losing her sight and hearing. She was also fearful of the future because she was losing control of the things that were happening in her body. M. expressed her feelings and said 'my mind frightened me very much but I still live in hope'.

I often remained for half an hour, spending most of the time listening to her story and giving the massage for her legs. During the massage she talked much more freely, talking of her past life as a happy active person who loved her country and she would like to speak to her son in Uganda because 'I don't have time left, I need to make phone call now'. She had been in touch then with her eldest son, he knew she was ill but not was told not to tell the younger boys. She made this phone call to her son and four days later she died peacefully . During these times I hoped I was helping towards her maintaining her quality of life. I was trying to give her as good a quality of time as possible. She shared with me how important time is. I felt she needed to talk through the whole experience and recognised her unspoken need for support and confidentiality. I believe this AIDS patient needed a compassionate and sympathetic listener, who would spend time in building a relationship that could support her through the AIDS experience.

Case History 2

J. was a very courageous lady in her late forties, married with two sons, aged 18 and 17 years. She had been diagnosed six years previously and she had coped well with her metastatic breast cancer causing widespread bone pain. During her stay in the local hospice for symptom control, her bone pain was eventually well controlled by medication, but she became low in mood, tearful and panicky. Depression was treated with anti-depressants (amitriptyline) and she was started on a tricyclical (parsteline) to help her sleep and lift her mood.

She expressed her main fear which was that of recurrence because the doctor explained as gently as possible to J. and her husband that her disease had not only returned but was widespread throughout her body. She had many questions such as 'How soon would she die?' and 'would the pain become unbearable?' She was tearful and talking about the sadness at having to leave her husband and two boys. She also spoke about her deteriorating condition, losing her independence and the indignity of needing help to use the commode.

She had been rather an anxious woman, and had symptoms of depression in early adult life. During her illness she was to experience great physical, psychological, emotional and spiritual pain. She described to me her fear and apprehensiveness for the future.

A psychiatric referral was made and her mood improved greatly. She was encouraged to attend the Day Centre and she had been doing some painting, and rehabilitation for her consisted of learning relaxation techniques which she enjoyed. She was working on the painting and she said that 'It is so good to come somewhere where I can try something new and forget my illness. Thank you for helping me to enjoy life again.' She had enjoyed painting and her paintings were around her room. Time and again she remarked on how much she enjoyed this time in her life.

She had maintained very honest and open communication with her family and health professionals. Also extra social support was arranged with social workers and psychologists and physiotherapists and chaplain. Doctors and nurses were able to explain what was happening in terms that she was able to understand.

The information was given so that J. could use it to formulate her own thoughts and wishes rather than as explicit advice that she was encouraged to use in her life.
> 'Nurses always sit with me and when I need them, will be here with me, that is nice,
> that is really nice. Ask me first 'how do you feel?' then if I can't tell you, please still
> listen, don't go away.'

In this way her autonomy and rights as an individual were respected. While she is an extremely brave and realistic woman, she understandably needed much professional support and reassurance that appropriate care would be available when necessary. She lived on for six months after I met her. She went to bed and five hours later she died very peacefully.

Conclusion

Life-threatening illness care needs that extra something; the sensitivity and nuance of real sympathy with other human beings, understanding their world and meaning of their life, having an illness are part of that world and meaning.

"You matter because you are you. You matter to the last moment of your life, and we will do all we can to help you not only to die peacefully, but also to live until you die."

(12)

Saunders (1981) says that "an education is the key to the dissemination of new attitudes and knowledge throughout the nursing and medical establishments, in order that care for all dying patients should improve, no matter where they are cared for, at home or in hospital." She also believed that the hospice philosophy could be used in a variety of settings - the home, hospital, nursing homes and that it did not rely on a purpose-built building.

(13)

A little lady a week before her death said 'Three months ago I felt I wished to die because of increasing back ache and loss of dignity and loneliness but now my fear is all gone... I think I am ready... But please remember that my life belongs to me, those I love and those who love me.'

I believe that the challenge for medical education is to change our attitude. An approach which places respect for patients' autonomy as the highest priority for ethical healthcare will result in benefits and we will retain society's trust and confidence.

We have to take responsibility for our future. Over the last 50 years it was rebuilt in Japan. Now perhaps it is time for us to rebuild ourselves to face the future in palliative care. It's a new beginning.

References

1. World Health Organisation (1990) Cancer pain relief and palliative care. Technical Report Series 804. Geneva.
2. Department of Health (1995) A policy framework on commissioning cancer services. Calman Report.
3. Higginson I (1993) Palliative care: a review of past changes and future trends. Journal of Public Health Medicine Vol 15 No 1 3-8.
4. Glickman M (1996) Palliative care in the hospital setting. National Council for hospice and specialist palliative care services.
5. Sontag S (1991) Illness as metaphor AIDS and its metaphors. Penguin Book.
6. Webb P (1986) Issues that influence information giving in Europe. European Journal of Cancer Care, 5 Supplement 1 1-8.
7. Doyle D (1986) Palliative care: the management of far advanced illness. Croom Helm Books.
8. Malin C (1996) The special case of clinical trials. European Journal of Cancer Care, 5 Supplement 1 1-8.
9. Buckman R (1992) How to break bad news. Papermac.
10. The national cancer alliance (1996) Patient-centred cancer services "What patients say".
11. Grahm G (1996) Patient information as a necessary therapeutic intervention. European Journal of Cancer Care 5 Supplement 1.
12. Saunders C (1983) Living with dying. Oxford University Press.
13. Saunders C (1990) Hospice and palliative care. Edward Arnold.

Patients' Perceptions of Palliation in Japan

Keiko Hamaguchi , R.N.,OCNS [1], Yasuko Ishigaki, R.N. [1], Kunihiko Ishitani ,M.D.[2]

1 Department of Nursing and 2 Department of Internal Medicine, Higashi Sapporo Hospital, Higashi Sapporo 3-3-7-35, Shiroihi-ku , Sapporo, 003 Japan

SUMMARY. In 1996, a multicenter collaborative study of the home cancer care was conducted thoughout Japan. As of March 31, 1997, a total of 208 home care cancer patients had been included in this study. In almost all cases, the objective was palliative care. This can be interpreted as meaning that the patient group who desired home care or were being given home care had made clear their desire for palliation. The rate of notification of the true disease diagnosis was a high 60% in the case of home care cancer patients. In addition, the rate of notification was significantly higher 1) in the younger patient group than in the older patient group, 2) in the patient group with a spouse than without a spouse, 3) in the patient group which received chemotherapy , 4) in the patient group which desired to continue home care. On the other hand , the patient's desire to continue home care at the time of starting home care showed correlations with 1) the relationship between the patient and the medical care personnel, 2) the patient's anxiety, and 3) the family's desire to continue home care. After 8 weeks of home care, significant correlations were found between patient's desire to continue home care and 1) the patient's satisfaction, 2) the relationship between the patient and the family, 3) the family's satisfaction, 4) the family's desire to continue home care. It is concluded that telling the truth improved patient's satisfaction in palliative care.

KEY WORDS: patient' perception, palliative care, home cancer care, notification of true diagnosis

INTRODUCTION

During last decade, the importance of palliative care for advanced cancer patients has been significantly addressed in Japan. The keys to improve the quality of palliative care are   1) to assess comprehensively patients' symptoms (physical and psychological),   2) to enhance the caregivers' expertise,   3) to care for patients and their families in a multidisciplinary fashion,   4) to improve patients' understanding of their disease through education and communication with patients and their families.

In Japan, cancer has been the number one cause of death since 1981. In 1996, malignancies were the cause of death in 30.3% of all deaths in Japan [1]. In recent years, cancer has come to be looked upon as a chronic disease, and today many people continue to live with cancer. In spite of these changes, even today a diagnosis of "cancer" carries with it a strong image of a disease which threatens one's life, that is cancer equals death. It can be imagined that patients' perceptions are probably influenced by what they know about their disease. We will discuss about this aspect of the treatment of cancer patients in Japan today.

STATUS OF NOTIFICATION OF DIAGNOSIS, SELECTION OF THERAPY AND SITE OF TREATMENT IN JAPAN

Status of notification of diagnosis in Japan

To date, almost no national surveys have been conducted in Japan with regard to the actual status of notification of patients that they have been diagnosed as having cancer. However, in 1994, the Ministry of Health and Welfare published the results of a survey of approximately one thousand six hundred surviving family members of deceased cancer patients, and the data indicated that 20.2% of the patients knew the true diagnosis of their disease, while another 44% had guessed the true diagnosis[2]. Compared with the findings of a 1992 survey, the percentage of patients knowing the true diagnosis has been increasing gradually. In addition, there are now some hospitals and doctors who have adopted a policy of informing almost all cancer patients of their true disease diagnosis. It indicate attitudes in Japan have shifted with regard to disclosing information to patients about their own diagnosis.

Status of explanation given to patients regarding their disease

With regard to the status of the explanation the cancer patients had received about their disease and diagnosis, among the patients who "knew the true diagnosis," the largest category was "given a detailed explanation." On the other hand, in the patient groups of "guessed true diagnosis" and "did not know the true diagnosis," about 40-50% each had "not been given any explanation." [2] When we consider palliation, it can be surmised that the first step is the patients' knowing whether or not their disease can be cured, or whether it will be difficult to cure. If a patient is not given an explanation regarding the disease diagnosis and his or her status and is placed in a position of uncertainty, it will be very difficult for the patient to make important decisions affecting his or her life, including the method and site of treatment.

Attitudes of out patients and doctors toward notification

In 1996, a survey of outpatients was conducted at 7 medical institutions around Japan, including cancer centers[3]. More than 80% of the patients expressed a desire to be told about the therapeutic method, and the efficacy and side effects of the therapy. However, only 66% said they "wanted to know if they had cancer." In addition, in the younger patient group, significantly high percentages gave a reply of "want to know" with regard to the "explanation of the prognosis" and a reply of "I want to decide for myself" in relation to the question of the "final decision of therapy." These desires regarding the handling of the disease also showed a significant correlation with the level of education of the patient. No gender-based differences were found.

A survey was also made of the opposite side of the patient-doctor relationship, that is, the doctors (n=932), with regard to the question of notification of cancer patients about their disease. Only 7% of the doctors said they "would like to explain the true health status, even if not hopeful of cure." On the other hand, most of the doctors took a position of case-by-case decision of what to do, answering that they "think it is better to explain the true health status, whenever possible" or "think explanation of the true health status should be given only after careful consideration." In addition, there were many doctors who said they favored notification if the prognosis was good, but not if the likelihood of cure was low [4]. It can be surmised that this approach is good since it takes into consideration the individual circumstances and QOL of the patient, but on the other hand the decision will be strongly influenced by the doctor's personal philosophy.

Actual status of selection of therapy and site of treatment

It can be surmised that the degree of explanation of the diagnosis and disease condition given to the patient influences the patient's selection of the therapy and the site of treatment.

The Ministry of Health and Welfare survey also looked into the question of—once it was realized that the patient would probably die—who actually selected the treatment to be administered[2].

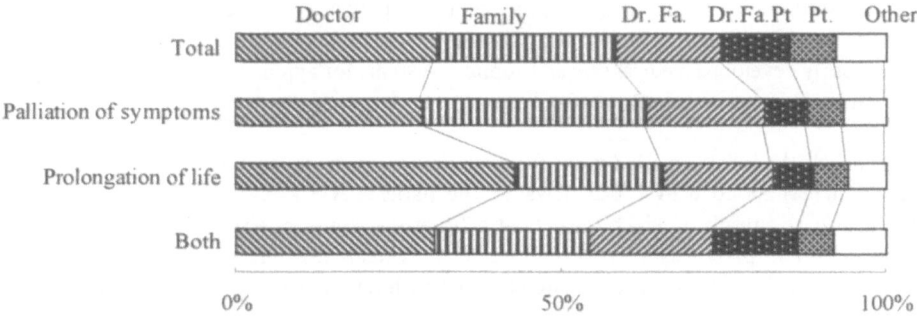

Fig. 1. Person(s) who considered and requested medical treatment, as function of the desired objective of the treatment (the Ministry of Health and Welfare survey)

The selection was made by the patient, doctor and family 9.4% of the time and 6.8% of the time by the patient, whereas the patient was not involved in the decision 70% of the time [Fig. 1] .

Furthermore, when the data were broken down as a function of the objective of the desired therapy, in the case of "prolongation of life," the decision of the therapy was about 40% made by the doctor. However, there is a question of what "prolongation of life" really means. That is, radical therapy will not necessarily prolong life, and conversely, palliative therapy aimed at alleviating symptoms may prolong life. Thus, there is a problem with the survey in relation to its terminology and methodology. In addition, it can be surmised that the true, behind-the-scenes role of the patient might be varied in cases where it is said that "the decision of the therapy was left up to the doctor." That is, it may be that the patient knew what the doctor's decision was going to be, did not disagree with it and thus let the doctor make that decision, or it may be that the patient truly left the decision entirely up to the doctor. It is necessary to distinguish between these situations, because the patients' perception are different. The first situation is actually a case of the patient's making the decision himself or herself.

With regard to the place of treatment desired by the patients and their families, roughly equal percentages of patients—about 45%—hoped for hospitalization and for outpatient care or treatment at home. The largest percentage of the families expressed a desire that the patient be hospitalized. On the other hand, when the actual site of treatment was analyzed as a function of the duration of the treatment, it is seen that 22.3% of the cancer patients were continually hospitalized for the last 6 months before death. Hospitalization during the last month of life was the overwhelming case, at 71% [2] .

Background factors thought to influence notification and palliative therapy

It can be said that the current situation in Japan with regard to notification of patients of the diagnosis of their disease is similar to the situation that existed in the United States in the 1960s. Various background factors can be thought to influence notification and palliation (Table 1).

Table 1. Background factors thought to influence notification and palliation
1. National Characteristics of Japanese
    Family-oriented lifestyle
    Mutual dependence
2. Paternalism of health care workers
3. Problems of medical care cost
    Hospitalization is the cheapest approach for the patient
4. Problems of health care system
    Poorly developed medical care and support systems for application
    at home , in intermediate, nursing home

They include the following. (1) Firstly the family are given an explanation of the patient's disease and often hesitate to deliver bad news to the patient. A society with a feeling of mutual dependence, as a result of which the patient believes that someone else will look after himself or herself. (2) The paternalism in the medical care system. (3) The patients who know their diagnosis are more likely choose the site of their health care. A current problem of high costs for medical care in Japan, yet the patient's share of the total cost is smaller when he or she is hospitalized. And (4), there has been little development of out-patient support systems, such as home care, and it is difficult for advanced cancer patient to be treated except in hospital.

PERCEPTION OF ADVANCED CANCER PATIENTS BEING TREATED AT HOME

From January of 1996, the Japanese Foundation for Multidisciplinary Treatment of Cancer initiated a multicenter collaborative research of the home cancer care. The objectives of this research are (1) to investigate the degree of satisfaction of the home care patient and his or her family with the care at home, and the factors influencing that degree of satisfaction, (2) to elucidate the roles and the status of cooperation between the various health care providers involved in the home care, and (3) to design a rational and effective system for home cancer care. The protocol for this study anticipated that high-technology home care and hospice home care would be provided, but in the end we found that in almost all cases the objective was palliative care. This can be interpreted as meaning that the patient group who desired home care or were being given home care had made clear their desire for palliation.

Research methods

The 22 institutions are participating in this nationwide research project. The individual background of patients, such as diagnosis, history, economical condition, and patient and family satisfaction, physical and psychosocial condition, activity of daily living (ADL) ,etc., including 34 items using a simple 4-grade scale were assessed. Their assessments were performed at the time of transfer to home care, and then every 2 weeks thereafter, continuing until the patient dies at home or is readmitted to the hospital.

Background characteristics of patients

As of March 31, 1997, a total of 208 home care cancer patients had been included in this study. They consisted of 97 males and 111 females. The mean age was 67.0 years, with a range of 9 to 96 years. The greatest number of patients were in their 70s: 32.7%. The most common type of malignancy was digestive tract cancers, in 141 patients, or 67.8% of the total. In addition, the outcome of the switch to home care has been death at home for 82 patients, and a return to the hospital for 115 patients (Table 2).

Table 2.   Background Characteristics of Patients

Numbers of Subject:	208 (Male 97 , Female 111)
Mean Age	: 67.0 (Range ; 9-96, Median 68, SD13.9) ,
Cancer Site	: Digestive tract 141 (67.8%)
	Lung 29 (13.9%)
Outcome	: Death at Home 82 (39.4%)
	Readmission to Hospital 115 (55.3%)
Length of home care	: 51.6±62.4 (Median ; 31days, Range ; 1 - 418)

Status of notification of true diagnosis

Over fifty-nine percent of the home care patients "knew the true diagnosis" of their disease, while 24% "did not know the true diagnosis" because they had not been told. Thus, the percentage of home care cancer patients covered by this national survey who had been notified of the true diagnosis was high.

Relationship between the age and notification of true diagnosis

Analysis of the relationship between the age of the patient and notification of the true diagnosis showed that the younger patients had the highest rate of notification: 84% for patients younger than 50 years of age. Conversely, the lowest rate of notification was 24% in the patients in their 80s, and the difference between the older patients group and the younger patients group was statistically significant. When the total patients were divided into 2 groups with 70 years as the cut-off, the 69-and- younger group showed a high percentage of cases who knew the true

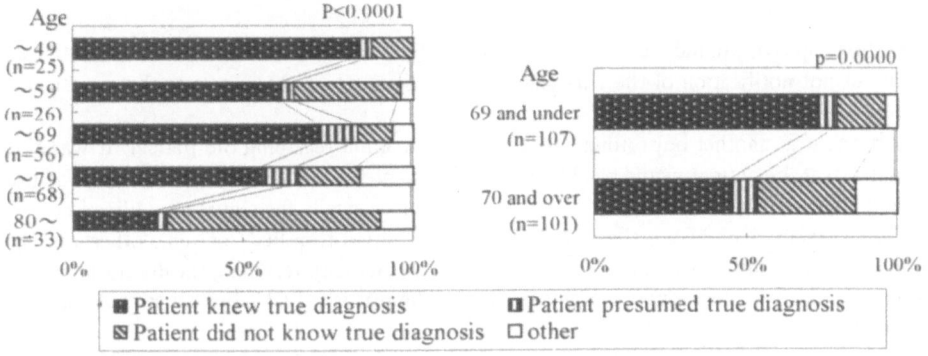

Fig. 2.   Relationship between the age and notification of true diagnosis

diagnosis, while the 70-and-older group had a high percentage of cases who did not know the true diagnosis. The difference between these two groups was statistically significant (Fig 2). This finding shows that, even if they are not notified of their true diagnosis, the older patients are transferred to home care because palliation is considered to be feasible. However, it can be surmised that there is a possibility that these older patients become aware that the end of their life is near in view of the aging phenomenon.

Relationship between patient's gender or existence of a spouse and notification of true diagnosis

There has been a tendency for the rate of notification to be lower for female cancer patients than for males. But it is not statistically significant(Fig 3). There has been a tendency for the rate of

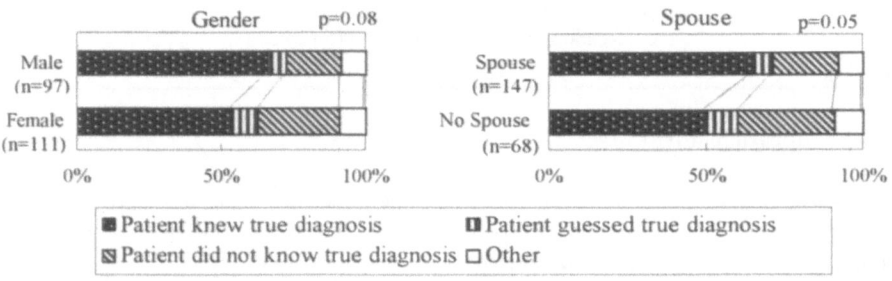

Fig. 3. Relationship between patient gender or existence of a spouse and notification of true diagnosis

notification to be higher in the patient group with a spouse compared to the group without a spouse (Fig. 3) . No correlation was found between notification and the number household members. These findings indicate that the spouse is being considered to be a key person by the doctor.

Relationships between number of times of admission and type of treatment unit and notification of true diagnosis

No relationship was found between the number of times of admission to the hospital and whether or not notification of the true diagnosis was given (Fig. 4). Each time that a patient is admitted to
the hospital, it is another opportunity to collect information regarding the patient. It was thus speculated that the patient would be able to gain an accurate understanding of his or her condition. However, these survey results indicate that there was no change in the status of notification.
In addition, comparison of whether the patient was admitted to a PCU or some other unit also did not reveal any difference in the understanding of the patients regarding the diagnosis of their disease (Fig.4). Even among patients who wanted to be put in a PCU, there were patients who did not know the true diagnosis.

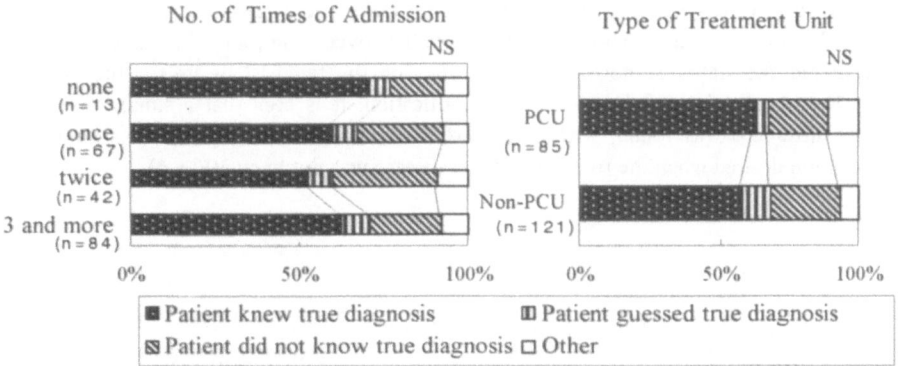

Fig. 4. Relationships between number of times of admission and type of treatment unit and notification of true diagnosis

Relationship between the type of treatment and notification of true diagnosis

Many of the patients in the group administered chemotherapy were given notification, and there was a statistically significant difference with the patient group not receiving chemotherapy (Fig.5).

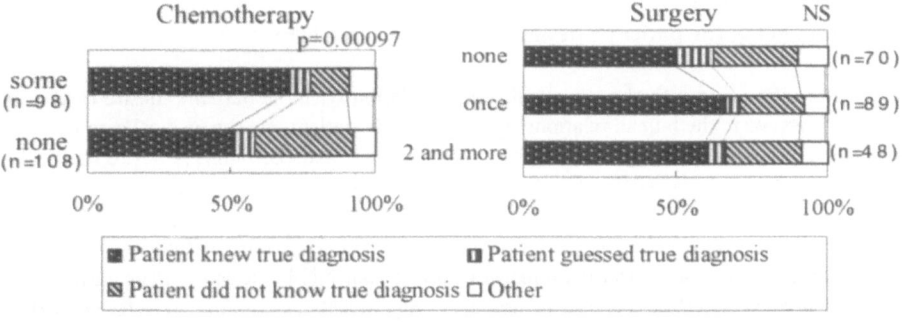

Fig. 5. Relationship between the type of treatment and notification of true diagnosis

On the other hand, surgery did not show any correlation with notification. However, it should be noted that it is unclear whether or not notification was carried out before the treatment was administered.

Finally, no correlation was found between notification and either patient satisfaction, or the psychological state of the patient, such as anxiety, the physical symptoms.

Desire to continue home care

It surmised that the patient's desire to continue home care, which reflects the patient's perception of the palliation. This question had 4 possible answers: "return to hospital," "return to hospital, if possible," "continue home care, if possible" and "continue home care until death." There was a tendency for patients who had been told the true diagnosis of their disease to desire

220

to continue home care, whereas patients who did not know the diagnosis or their disease status desired to be hospitalized. A correlation was found between the patient's desire to continue home care and the status of notification. The data on the families' desire for the patient to continue home care relative to the status of notification. It is seen that a similar statistically significant difference was found, with home care favored when the diagnosis was known, and hospitalization desired when the true diagnosis or disease was not known(Fig. 6).

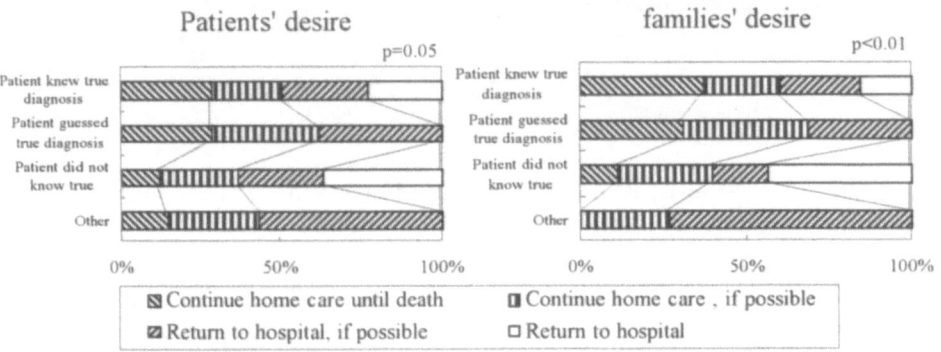

Fig. 6. Relationship between patients' and families' desire to continue home care and notification of true diagnosis

Factors influencing the patient's desire to continue home care

Several factors were found to show a significant correlation with the patients' desire to continue home care. They were the human relationship between the patient and the medical care personnel (that is, a relationship of trust), the anxiety of the patient, and the family's desire to continue home care.

During the 8-week period after the start of home care, the correlation coefficients compiled for the factors found to be related to the patient's desire to continue home care. In the patient group aged less than 70 years, after 8 weeks of home care significant correlations were found with the family's desire for continued home care, the patient's satisfaction, the family's satisfaction and the relationship between the patient and the family (Table 3). It surmised that a high level of satisfaction on the part of the caregiver is an important factor in support of continuation of home care of the cancer patient. On the other hand, there are no factors showing a significant correlation.

Table 3. Factors influencing the patient's desire to continue home care

Patient group aged less than 70 years	Start of home care	2 weeks	4 weeks	6 weeks	8 weeks
The number of family caregivers	0.509	0.274	0.241	0.361	0.390
Family's desire for continued home care	0.401	0.571	0.578	0.639	0.655
Patient's satisfaction	-0.272	-0.070	-0.170	-0.290	-0.680
Family's satisfaction	-	0.004	-0.020	0.008	-0.550
Human relationship between Patient and Family	0.473	0.394	0.209	0.333	0.515

CONCLUSION

The following points summarise the findings (Table 4).

Table 4   Summary
Patient' perception would be related to
· aging
· level of education of the patient
· in the patient group which received chemotherapy
· the patient's desire to continue home care
Patient's desire to continue home care would be related to
· the patient's satisfaction and psychosocial condition
· the family's satisfaction and desire to continue home care

Patient' perception, the status of notification of the diagnosis would be related to aging and level of education of the patient, in the patient group which received chemotherapy, and, the patient's desire to continue home care. In addition, the patient's desire for home care showed correlations with the patient's satisfaction, psychological condition, the family's satisfaction ,the family's desire for continued home care, and the relationship between the patient and the family.

Future Topics

The following topics need to be investigated in future of advanced cancer patients.
1. Who influences the patient's perception of home care?
2. Education of medical care personnel, including implementation of evidence-based medicine.
3. Education of patients, their families and the general population.

The number of oncologists and oncology nurses is still small in Japan. Instead, most medical care personnel are involved in the administration of cancer treatment. It can be surmised that, if there were an increase in the number of specialists handling cancer therapy, there would be development of various aspects of psychosocial support, such as psycho-oncology, and changes would occur in relation to notification of patients of the true diagnosis of their disease and also in the methods of treatment. There would also be development of a specialty dealing with the patients' perceptions of their disease and treatment. Patients' perceptions are of course important, but so are the perceptions of palliation held by medical care personnel, and for this reason greater education of medical care personnel, including implementation of evidence-based medicine is needed. Oncologists are still rare in Japan, and recognition of special nursing requirements within the specialty of oncology has just begun to take hold. The treatment of cancer patients is essentially being carried out on a trial-and-error basis by a full range of medical care personnel. We conclude that it is necessary for Japan to develop specialists in cancer therapy.

REFERENCES

1. Summary of Vital statistics, MINISTRY OF HEALTH AND WELFARE , http ://www.

mhw.   go.jp / english / database / index.html, 1997.10.
2. Statistics and Information department, minister's secretariat, MINISTRY OF HEALTH AND WELFARE: Report on the socioeconomic survey of vital statistics; The medical treatment for the terminally ill patient FY 1994.
3. Mitsuru Hisata, Nobuo Okazaki, Ichiro Kai, Yasushi Nomura, Hideyuki Saeki., Yasunosuke Sakata, Eiichi Nagura, Yoko Emukai, Kenjiro Tanemura, Jun Hiraoka , Kunihiko Ishitani (1996) , Attitudes of Outpatients toward Informed Consent in Cancer Treatment, J. Jpn Soc Cancer Ther. 31(3):171-185
4. Tomomi Hayashi(1996), Japanese Mind and Notification of Cancer Diagnosis (in Japanese) , Japan Cancer Pathophisics and Therapy Study QOL Group

Patient Education and Ethics

Makoto Aoki

Office of Medical Information, AIDS Clinical Center, International Medical Center of Japan.
1-21-1, Toyama, Shinjuku-ku, Tokyo, 162, Japan

INTRODUCTION

Conventional approach in palliative medicine lead mainly by physicians has been almost always in the context of physical paradigm. There, while physical problems such as pain or dyspnea was well taken care of or at least was in the list of medical problems in the chart, fears and loneliness surrounding the terminally ill were often neglected or taken as "natural" or inevitable suffering by healthcare team. But three papers presented at the last session of the symposium challenges this kind of conventional approaches.

The first paper, " Complementary and Alternative Medicine" , presented by Dr. Stephen C. Schimpf, Executive Vice President, the University of Maryland Medical System, shed light on how much money is actually being spent for complementary and alternative medicine in the United States indicating a strong need for and belief in such kind of approaches. (More than $13 billion per year is spent in the United States, with much of that uninsured and paid in cash and credit card payments and without knowledge of the patient's physician.) These approaches include diet, exercise, stress reduction methodologies, acupuncture, acupressure, meditation, herbal medicine, and so on. Most of the dying patients are not trying to eradicate the fatal illness by complementary and alternative approaches. Instead, they are seeking comfort, acceptance by family, colleague, or medical personal which are significant part of quality of life (QOL). " Patients with diseases like cancer and AIDS are understandably frightened; They are not satisfied with an approach by their physicians that focuses on technology yet is lacking in empathy, listening and true attention to supportive care. Today, as a result, patients visit alternative practitioners without informing their doctor." says Dr. Schimpf. He states that even if physicians, themselves, cannot or will not devote adequate attention to supportive care measures, it is critical that the overall health care team is organized in a fashion to do so. He also educated us how much improvement in QOL could be brought in by complementary and alternative approaches. This improvement in some of complementary and alternative medicine was even statistically significant by scientific analysis. Despite apparent integrity of the study designs, physician seem able to undermine or largely ignored this body of data. We should also focus not only on the statistically significant improvement in physical condition such as pain or dyspnea with those complementary and alternative approach but also on the fact that people working in this field are actually spending more time with patients. Perhaps the attraction in these approaches for patients is that they targeted dimensions of well being which go beyond the strictly physical paradigm. Dr. Schimpf closed his paper with following remarks. " The exact role of complementary and alternative medicine in cancer or AIDS supportive care is unclear, but it is apparent that cancer patients seek out holistic approaches and look to these techniques and practitioners as one aspect of holistic care. Hence, at minimum, Oncologist and AIDS physicians must become aware and knowledgeable."

The second paper, " Support with Information, Education and Counseling in Patients with Advanced cancer and AIDS " was presented by Ms. Mayumi Abe whose experience in palliative care in both Japan as well as in England put her on excellent position to compare different palliative care provided in different cultural background. She works now in St. Christopher's Hospice, London, UK where she takes care of patients with terminal cancer and HIV related condition. (There has been no hospice in Japan which has routinely accepted patients with HIV diseases.) While some discussion regarding the cultural difference between Japan and Western medical practices were outlined, it appeared that what we have in common may outweigh our differences. She also helped us to go back to the bedside of patients -- a position that we should never stay far from. Further more she also reminded us that palliative care is not confined to last days of life, but speaks to a holistic approach which can be utilized and applied to a broad variety of patients.

The third paper " Patient's Perception of Palliation " presented by Ms.Keiko Hamaguchi from Department of Nursing, Higashi Sapporo Hospital, Sapporo, Japan, discussed the issue of truth telling and disclosure of information to patients with cancer. In Japan, it appears that the configuration of decision-making consisting of doctors, families and patients is most heavily weighed towards doctors then families rather than towards patients first. The practice of truth telling and disclosure of information to patients occured in North America over the last 30 years. Along with the changing practices in North America has been a transition which has seen physicians moving from a paternalistic stance to more collaborative effort in which their patients are seen as equal partners. The third paper also indicated that younger patients (less than 69 year old) experienced more satisfaction with truth telling and disclosure of information compared with older patients (more than 70 year old).

Dr. Harvey M. Chochinov, from Department of Psychiatry, the University of Manitoba , who was my co-chair of this last session and was great help in preparation of this summary, concludes this session with following messages. " This symposium was not merely a one-way street in which Westerners attempted to show their Japanese hosts how to do palliative care, but rather a two-way street in which a both hosts and guests taught and learned a great deal from one another."

KEY WORD INDEX